The
Lazy Girl's Guide
to **a Blissful**
Pregnancy

Anita Naik is a freelance writer, author and columnist. She specialises in parenting, pregnancy, and lifestyle issues and writes regularly for a variety of magazines including *Glamour*, *Red* and *Prima Baby*, as well as the pregnancy and parenting site www.bounty.com, and MIDIRS (Midwives Information and Resource Service). She is also the author of over forty books and was previously the agony aunt on *Just17*, *Closer* and *TV Quick* magazines. Anita is currently the agony aunt on *Teen Now* and the Bebo sponsored page, Lady Lounge. For more information go to www.anitanaik.co.uk.

Anita is also the author of:
The Lazy Girl's Guide to Beauty
The Lazy Girl's Guide to Good Health
The Lazy Girl's Guide to Good Sex
The Lazy Girl's Guide to a Fabulous Body
The Lazy Girl's Party Guide
The Lazy Girl's Guide to Men
The Lazy Girl's Guide to Success
The Lazy Girl's Guide to Green Living
The Lazy Girl's Guide to the High Life on a Budget
Think Yourself Gorgeous
Babe Bible
The New You
Pocket Babe
Kitchen Table Tycoon

The
Lazy Girl's Guide
to a Blissful
Pregnancy

Anita Naik

piatkus

PIATKUS

First published in Great Britain in 2011 by Piatkus

Copyright © 2011 by Anita Naik

The moral right of the author has been asserted.

All rights reserved.
No part of this publication may be reproduced, stored in a retrieval system,
or transmitted in any form or by any means, without the prior permission
in writing of the publisher, nor be otherwise circulated in any form of
binding or cover other than that in which it is published and without a
similar condition including this condition being imposed on the subsequent
purchaser.

A CIP catalogue record for this book
is available from the British Library.

ISBN 978-0-7499-5321-8

Typeset in Minion by Phoenix Photosetting, Chatham, Kent
Printed and bound in Great Britain by CPI Mackays, Chatham ME5 8TD
Illustrations by Anna Hymas, New Division

Piatkus
An imprint of
Little, Brown Book Group
100 Victoria Embankment
London EC4Y 0DY

An Hachette UK Company
www.hachette.co.uk

www.piatkus.co.uk

For Bella, Joe and Jimmy – who was but a bump
during the making of this book

While all the nutrients and dietary changes referred to in this book have been proven safe, those seeking help for specific medical conditions are advised to consult a qualified nutritional therapist, doctor or equivalent health professional. The recommendations given in this book are solely intended as education and information and should not be taken as medical advice. Neither the authors nor the publisher accept liability for readers who choose to self-prescribe.

Contents

Acknowledgements

With thanks to all the mums and mum-to-be lazy girls who, despite being so frantic and time starved, sent me their thoughts, words of wisdom, expert advice and funny anecdotes on life being pregnant and beyond.

Introduction

For many of us life is way too busy and stressful. Most of the time we feel horribly time starved as if we were on a speeded up treadmill rushing from A to B, trying to keep everyone happy. Factor into this a pregnancy, the whole idea of labour and life after birth and all that comes with it, and it's likely that you'll feel as if you're going crazy.

When I was pregnant the first time around, the weeks went by in a blur of relentless activity, where I struggled to mix my everyday life with my social life and my new pregnant life. As a result, my idea of a blissful and informed pregnancy where I got to savour what was happening and indulge myself never really happened. Most of the time, like so many pregnant women, I wasn't lying on a sofa relaxing, but rushing about trying to fit in appointments and work deadlines.

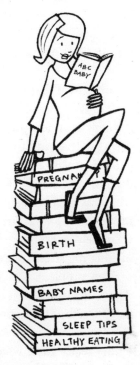

Working right up to the week of my daughter's delivery, I lived to regret my decision not to relax and let go of life's reins for nine months. Why? Well, because once my daughter came along, the true meaning of being busy came into full force. I wished then that I had spent more time lying back being lazy and enjoying what was happening. Next time I swore it would be different, except that I am now pregnant for the second time, with a three year old in tow and a business to run, meaning that most of the time being lazy and relaxed is the furthest thing from my mind.

If you feel like this, then rest assured that you're not alone. Studies show that only about 1 per cent of us can afford to give up work when we get pregnant and to erase our lives of a schedule so that we can get to grips and focus on what's happening to us. This means that 99 per cent of us have to struggle to find the time to work out what pregnancy is all about while trying to run our lives. Mostly, this rightly means focusing on the medical and health stuff, which is a shame because, as you may already be discovering, this isn't the only stuff that irks and worries us during pregnancy.

It's also the reason why most of us end up wading through countless pregnancy books, magazines and websites desperately trying to find solutions to everything from the painful stuff to the weird stuff and the everyday stuff that's driving us crazy. In fact, so determined was I to find out what was happening to my body and mind – not to mention my spreading waistline and fluctuating moods – that I read absolutely everything I could get my hands on, thereby making my stressful life even more stress filled.

The problem was that some of this information was depressing, some of it overly complicated and some just too loaded with information to make much sense. And most of the time I couldn't even find the answer I was looking for. I now realise that what I needed was not 1,000 books on pregnancy, but one book that condensed all the information into a perfect lazy guide that would tell me a 1,000 different things about being pregnant. That's 1,000 things about the worries a midwife can't always help you with – anxieties and annoyances, such as:

- Why am I in a bad mood all the time?
- How will I cope financially?
- Why do I look fat and not pregnant?
- What if I hate being a mum?
- Why do other pregnant women glow gorgeously while I look like I have been dragged through a hedge backwards?
- How come I've forgotten how to do my work/get dressed/ drive properly?

Hence, the creation of *The Lazy Girl's Guide to a Blissful Pregnancy*! It's a lazy girl's guide because being pregnant, whether for the first time or the fourth time, means that even though you are pregnant, life still has to go on. That's your social life, work life and everything else in your life, which equals a hugely busy time when you should be finding more time to relax and be lazy. And it's about a blissful pregnancy, because that's what most of us are looking for: a pregnancy with more bliss, and less stress and irritation all round.

As a result, this book is crammed full of helpful and calming advice from experts, other pregnant women and mums, as well as specialists in the field of exercise, relationships, styling and beauty. My aim is not only to help smooth the pregnancy path for you but also to help lighten your load just a little.

Better still, the book is designed in such a way that if you are extremely lazy (busy or stressed, for that matter), you can read it on a dip-in/dip-out basis, focusing on what's bothering you right now, or you can read it from cover to cover, or simply read the glossary in Chapter 8 (although I wouldn't recommend doing only that).

Whichever route you take, rest assured that somewhere in here will be an answer to your lifestyle query/worry/fear/irk, as well as tips on how to cope and enjoy being pregnant, and even what to do when it all gets too much for you.

Remember being pregnant is something to be enjoyed, even if you don't like the process all that much, so it's worth doing your best to iron out all those niggling parts about body worries, mood swings and complicated birth instructions. After all, it's going to be more than worth it in the end.

PS: Baby is referred to as 'him' or 'her' in alternate sections of this book for ease of reading, although the book relates to all babies equally.

CHAPTER ONE

So you're pregnant

Yippee, I'm pregnant! Discovering that you're pregnant is right up there with some of life's greatest highs. In an instant you'll feel as if you've climbed Everest, won an Oscar and zipped yourself into a size 8 pair of jeans all at once. The problem is that once the initial euphoria of finding out has passed, you're likely to be left feeling a jumble of nerves, and probably stuffed to the brim with what-ifs and dilemmas, such as who to tell and when?

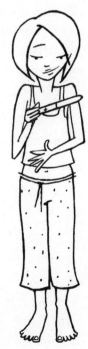

What next?

The fact is that no one ever really tells you what you ought to do once you find out you are pregnant. You know you have to see a doctor at some point and tell people such as friends, family and work, but what on earth do you do in the meantime?

tip

Pregnancy tests are *the* best way to work out if you're pregnant or not. But if you do one in a rush, or don't read the instructions, it is all too easy to get a false negative: the test says you're not pregnant but you actually are. Help yourself by not testing too early, and reading the instructions carefully.

Who to tell?

Although there are many thoughts on who you should tell and when, with many people leaning towards the don't-mention-a-thing-till-you're-12-weeks because of the risk of miscarriage, in truth it is entirely up to you. Plenty of people spill the beans early, either because they are so excited that they can't keep it in or because they want to tell friends and family in case they do have a miscarriage.

"The first time round I told everyone at five weeks, from my mum to my work colleagues even the postman. I just couldn't keep the secret in."

Sam, 33

Of course, there is a whole realm of annoying people you shouldn't tell. The first and foremost is the superstitious friend/family member who will greet your good news with the words: 'Oh aren't you afraid you'll jinx things by telling everyone so early?'

Not only can you not jinx things by saying you are pregnant but also you can't bring on a miscarriage by talking about your pregnancy or feeling positive about it. Do what feels right for you. If you want to post your news on Twitter, then go for it, and if you want to keep it quiet for six months, that's your right too.

The second most annoying person to tell is the person who says, 'Oh I knew already. I could tell because you look pregnant/bigger/seemed so moody.' The reality is that they can't tell and are just trying to get one up on you.

And perhaps the most irritating person of all to tell is the Mumzilla – the friend/family member who lives for pregnancy and children and who will greet your news with the words, 'Right, well what you have to do is …' and carry on telling you what to do (and putting you in a panic) for the whole nine months.

Apart from these people, tell anyone, but do think very carefully before you bring it up at work. Although your boss can't fire you for being pregnant, or make you redundant because of your pregnancy (in all EU countries, Australia, New Zealand and North America you are protected when you are pregnant), the advice is to stay quiet. This is because the moment you mention you're pregnant, colleagues and your boss will start planning for your maternity leave and asking you questions that you won't yet know the answers to, such as: 'How long are you taking off?' 'Are you going to come back?' 'Will you be a working mother?' All these questions can be stressful when you haven't even got to grips with what it means to be pregnant yet.

What to do now?

There are plenty of things that you should be doing right from the moment you find out you are pregnant. This is because the most crucial part of your baby's development takes place in what's known as the first trimester (the first 12 weeks). So, how you treat your body, what you eat and the bad habits you ditch at this time will all affect your growing child.

Firstly, ditch the hard drinking and smoking. Depending on which country you live in, the advice on drinking varies, but what is certain is that alcohol in large amounts each week is detrimental to your baby's development. And you don't have to be a brain surgeon to realise the negative effects smoking has on your baby's development (see Chapter 2 for more on this). If you're finding it hard to give up, see your GP for specialised help and advice.

Secondly, make sure you are taking folic acid. In an ideal world you would have started to take it when you were trying to conceive, but don't worry if you haven't. Countless studies have shown that taking 400mcg of folic acid (sometimes called folate or vitamin B_9) daily prior to conception and during early pregnancy reduces the risk of serious neural tube defects such as spina bifida by up to 70 per cent. It's important to take these supplements until at least the twelfth week of your pregnancy, as folic acid plays an essential role in the development of your baby's brain, DNA and spinal cord.

fact

One in three pregnant women forget to take folic acid.

Finally, be prepared for mixed emotional feelings. Even if you were 100 per cent sure you wanted a baby, being surprised/shocked, scared, and even in denial, are normal reactions to a positive pregnancy test. Plus, once you start down the path of thinking about how you'll cope, how you'll manage with money, what to do about work and how it will change you as a person, it's all too easy to let being pregnant get to you. Rest assured that whatever you are feeling (negative or positive) has been experienced by countless other pregnant women.

"I cried for three days when I found out I was pregnant. We wanted a baby, but I kept worrying about how we'd cope. I worked a full week, and was the main earner, so we needed my wage, plus our flat was tiny and we had no savings. My boyfriend kept saying, 'It will be fine', and of course it was and still is, but the early days were so frightening."

Susie, 34

Help yourself by taking time to relax and not looking too far ahead. Pregnancy is overwhelming, and it's important to take each day of being pregnant a step at a time so that you can put your emotions and fears into perspective.

See your doctor

After telling your nearest and dearest, your doctor should be your first port of call once you are pregnant, and although he or she won't be eager to see you very early in your pregnancy it's vital that you make an appointment at some point between eight and ten weeks. This is because it takes time to get a hospital appointment (depending on where you live) and to arrange for any first-trimester screening tests, which usually need to be performed at around 12 weeks.

Be aware, however, that your initial appointment with your GP can feel like a bit of a let down, as doctors will rarely do another pregnancy test to see if you're pregnant but will simply take your word for it. Plus, it's too early to do anything exciting like listening for the baby's heart rate or seeing the baby on an ultrasound, but what a doctor will do is:

Talk about where you want to have your baby (don't worry, you can change your mind later). Your doctor should be able to advise you on the best hospital in your area as well as birth centres or a home birth. You will be asked now so that arrangements can be made for your antenatal midwife care to be at the same place where you will have your baby.

Advise you on your options of care. This means whether you'd prefer to see your GP and community midwives, or have midwife care within the hospital of your choice with an obstetrician. The former can be easier if you work and live locally; the latter can be easier if you work near the hospital.

Discuss your medical and pregnancy history. This is to pinpoint any potential problems that may need extra screening tests booked or to arrange a visit to the early-pregnancy unit for an early scan, which can usually be done around six or seven weeks of pregnancy (this usually occurs if you have had a past miscarriage or are at risk of miscarriage).

Work out your EDD (estimated delivery date). You can do the calculation yourself by subtracting three months from your last menstrual period (LMP), and then adding 7 days; for example:

If the first day of your LMP was 21 March, to work out your EDD you would have to take away three months (which takes you to 21 January) and then add seven days. This gives you an estimated due date of 28 January the following year.

However, bear in mind that this is an *estimate* and that only 5 per cent of women deliver on their EDD. Your date will also change as you have your various scans, which can give you a clearer idea of when you are due.

Talk about your pregnancy timeline. This is what is going to happen to you from here on in, in terms of the pregnancy, your baby's development, the length of your pregnancy (40 weeks) and the tests and scans you'll be offered.

What's the difference between screening tests and diagnostic tests?

A screening test estimates your risk of your baby having a disease or problem. So, an ultrasound is a screening test that allows you to 'see' your baby, and it also assesses the progress of your pregnancy and looks for possible abnormalities and problems; however, screening tests are only concerned with possible likelihoods, which means you might be told that there may be a problem when there is not, or be falsely reassured that all is well. Ultrasounds can, however, provide accurate information on: the number of babies you are carrying and the way that your baby is developing and the can detect some birth defects such as spina bifida.

A diagnostic test tells you for sure whether your baby has a problem or not, and these tests are accurate, because either a sample of tissue from the placenta or a sample of amniotic fluid is tested. Congenital heart defects and all chromosomal and genetic abnormalities can only be diagnosed with diagnostic tests such as chorionic villus sampling (CVS) and amniocentesis; however, they both carry a risk of miscarriage and so they tend to be offered only if your pregnancy is deemed to be at high risk. Talk to your midwife and doctor, and read up on the pros and cons of each test before you make your decision (see Resources for more information).

Advise you on vaccines, folic acid and your diet. Although this varies from country to country, on the whole you will be advised on what vaccines, if any, you need to take, as well as which vitamins are essential and which foods to stay away from.

fact

Your EDD is based on a rule that was developed in the mid 19th century (yes, that long ago!). It's calculated that the average gestational period of a pregnancy is 266 days (which equates to 38 weeks) from conception, or 280 days (40 weeks) from the first day of your LMP.

The early pregnancy bugbears

Early pregnancy is also, as you're probably discovering, a strange time. On the one hand it's madly joyful and euphoric and on the other it's tiring and exhausting. Although you probably knew you were going to feel ecstatic, it's unlikely anyone ever warned you about the pregnancy bugbears, the stuff that leaves you feeling exhausted and numb to the world in the early days.

I mention the above not because I want to rain on your pregnancy parade but because it pays to know that what's happening to you is not all in your head but a natural and normal part of being pregnant.

So, if you're currently feeling happy but weighed down by a whole host of early pregnancy symptoms, here's what you need to know.

1. Tender, swollen breasts

If you regularly get sore breasts around your period you'll know the feeling I'm talking about. Think swollen, tingly, sore, and/or a feeling that somehow your breasts are about to overflow your bra cups. Tender breasts like this are one of the first signs of pregnancy and occur thanks to rising levels of oestrogen and progesterone, which start to change breast tissue in readiness for milk for your growing baby. All of the above is why breast tenderness, soreness and even itchiness (this includes the nipple area) can start before you even know for sure you are pregnant.

Help yourself by wearing a well-fitting bra and having a hands-off policy until your breasts settle down.

2. Acute tiredness

This is not just your run-of-the-mill I've-had-an-exhausting-day tiredness, but the kind of tiredness you get when you're coming down with flu, where you imagine that if you close your eyes you'll fall asleep on the spot and not wake up for 24 hours!

This kind of fatigue happens because during early pregnancy your body diverts a large proportion of the energy that you usually use to start helping your baby to grow. The fact is, although you may just be discovering you are pregnant, the chances are you've been pregnant for a whole month or more, which means the baby will be in its embryonic period.

This in itself is a very important time of development, and although the embryo is still very small, it is growing rapidly, which means that the majority of your body's energy is given to your baby. The good news is that the worst of this fatigue goes away by the end of 12 weeks, although it will make a return in the last trimester because of the size of your baby.

Help yourself by learning to relax; take time out and generally just lie about on the sofa whenever you can. Going to bed much earlier than usual and not scheduling anything for a few weeks can also help to restore your energy and get you through the day.

3. An increased sense of smell

If you notice a heightened sense of smell, which makes everything from food to cigarette smoke smell vile, you could very well be pregnant. The 'official' thinking used to be that this increased sense of smell was your body's way of protecting the foetus from dangers to its development – that is, stopping you eating or breathing in something toxic; however, according to a 2005 study in the *International Journal of Obstetrics and Gynecology*, 'Pregnant women do not have olfactory processes different to non-pregnant women', meaning it's just another by-product of your pregnancy hormones.

Help yourself by carrying around something that smells good to you. That way you can clamp it to your nose whenever you smell something gut-wrenching. Try lavender oil, your favourite perfume or peppermints; if that doesn't work opt for fresh air as soon as possible.

4. Nausea and vomiting

Nausea, vomiting, that feeling that the room is swimming – also known as morning sickness – can hit you anytime of the day, beginning just a few short weeks into your pregnancy.

The culprit, as usual, is rising levels of hormones needed for your baby to grow.

Help yourself by eating little and often and keeping your meals plain and simple so that your stomach doesn't revolt on you.

fact

Around 75 per cent of women experience some kind of nausea and sickness in the first trimester.

5. Excessive peeing

Two to three weeks after conception (so basically when you don't yet realise you're pregnant) it's likely you'll feel the need to pee all the time. This urge is all down to the pregnancy hormone, human chorionic gonadotropin (HCG), which increases blood flow to your kidneys, helping them to more efficiently rid your body (and eventually, your baby's body) of waste.

Your growing uterus (yes, it's starting to grow already!) is also beginning to put some pressure on your bladder, leaving less storage space for urine and making you head for the toilet more often than you'd like. Although the need to pee constantly does go away around weeks 12–14, it makes a return the closer you get to your due date, once again down to the fact that your baby likes to tap dance on your bladder.

Help yourself by giving in to it – better out than in! Also, try to lean forwards when you pee, as this helps to empty the bladder completely, giving you a brief respite.

fact

You may notice that you need to get up to pee more often during the night. That's because when you lie down, some of the fluid that you retained in your legs and feet during the day makes its way back into your bloodstream and eventually into your bladder.

6. Insomnia

Pregnancy insomnia, especially in the first trimester, is very common. Mostly, it comes in the form of being unable to fall back to sleep after being awakened, probably from having to pee all the time. It's the result of stress and worry, but body heat can also be another problem, because in the early days of pregnancy you may find yourself suffering from hot flushes (and probably worrying that you're going through an early menopause). Again, this is normal and the result of an increased heart rate (your resting heart rate rises during pregnancy) as well as hormones. This is very much a first-trimester thing, but as your pregnancy progresses into the third trimester, your sleep will be disturbed as you fight to find a comfortable position, battling against restless legs and calf cramps (see page 14 for more on this).

Help yourself by keeping your room a little cooler than usual and winding down for 20 minutes before bed so that you feel more relaxed.

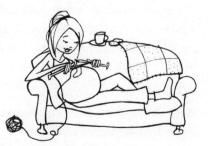

7. Restless leg syndrome

Over 25 per cent of pregnant women suffer from restless leg syndrome (RLS) – a horrible creepy-crawly, niggling feeling in your legs, that produces an overwhelming urge to move just as you're nodding off. Exhausting when it happens, it's a major source of sleep anxiety. If, however, you've been stretching your legs like a practised yogi with no sign of relief, stop right now; experts believe the cause is nutritional rather than physical.

Help yourself by taking an iron supplement (although seek advice from your doctor before you do this). One major US study shows that iron deficiency contributes to many cases of RLS. You may not have been diagnosed as clinically anaemic but your iron stores could still be low, as studies show 30 per cent of pregnant women don't get enough iron in their diet. Eat iron-rich foods (see page 77). Alternatively, try nettle tea. This has high levels of calcium, magnesium, iron, silica and potassium, all of which can help alleviate RLS. Avoid boiling the tea at high temperatures; just pour boiled water in and brew so you can retain the vitamin C.

8. Burping, wind and constipation

Pregnancy hormones will send your gastrointestinal tract on a rollercoaster ride. Cue lots of burping and bottom gas, not to mention constipation, as your intestines slow down and become sluggish. You may wonder what the heck is happening, but rest assured that it's just another sign of early pregnancy.

Help yourself by drinking plenty of water and eating fewer foods that are heavy to digest.

9. Dizziness

You're not imagining it, that dizzy and light-headed feeling is happening to you thanks to circulatory changes in the body. The trouble with feeling dizzy is that it can happen pretty much at any time, so when you're looking at a computer screen, or even driving, try to make time to rest, which can alleviate the feeling.

Help yourself by getting up slowly after you have been sitting or lying down. Eat regularly and avoid prolonged standing.

10. Backache

That's a lower backache in particular, the kind that sometimes happens before your period. It happens because your expanding uterus starts to move your centre of gravity and weakens your abdominal muscles, putting a strain on your back. There are two specific types of lower backache that tend to be linked to pregnancy: lumbar pain and posterior pelvic pain. First, you may feel lumber pain over and around your spine at waist level, and you may also experience nerve pain in your legs.

Help yourself by avoiding sitting or standing for long periods of time, and at the end of the day sit with your feet up for a while to relieve the pressure.

The second type of pain, posterior pelvic pain, is felt around the bottom and on the sides or the back of your thighs.

Help yourself by being careful about how you get off the sofa and bed, and limiting high-intensity exercise. Gentle stretching can also help here.

11. Weeping

Crying when you're not the crying type, or feeling yourself constantly moved to tears at an advert/cute baby/sad song on the radio, could be a sign that you are pregnant. Pregnancy hormones are to blame, once again, and this, mixed with anxiety about whether or not you are pregnant, tends to accelerate the crying process, especially around the sixth week of pregnancy.

Help yourself by finding out one way or another if you're pregnant or not.

A word about early pregnancy worries

The early days of pregnancy are also filled with a multitude of fears especially about miscarriage. Here's what you need to know to help put your mind at rest:

The risk of miscarriage

Although you won't want to think about this when you discover you are pregnant, it is worth knowing that 25 per cent of pregnancies end in a miscarriage. It's always a devastating experience, so it's important to know that miscarriages have nothing to do with what you do in the early stages of pregnancy. Getting drunk before you realise you are pregnant, drinking coffee, working overtime, lifting heavy stuff, exercising, sex and generally living your life as a normal non-pregnant person will not cause you to lose your baby.

fact

> Research shows that approximately 50 per cent of lost pregnancies have failed to develop normally, either due to chromosome or genetic problems, or because of structural (bodily) problems. There is no explanation for the remaining 50 per cent of cases.

If you do have three miscarriages in a row (which is rare) then you will be sent to a specialist who will determine if there is another problem, but on the whole, women who suffer one miscarriage do go on to have very healthy full-term pregnancies.

Bleeding in early pregnancy

The most common symptom of a miscarriage is bleeding from the vagina with abdominal pain, a bit like period pain (although some women get no symptoms at all). Not all bleeding means you are having a miscarriage. Half the women who bleed during pregnancy do not miscarry. This is because around the time of your period some pregnant women get a show of blood. Other women bleed in small spurts throughout their pregnancy, sometimes due to a small tear in the placenta wall. Others have what's known as a light implantation bleed, where they bleed as the egg implants into the endometrial wall.

What's important about bleeding is to seek medical advice as soon as possible. A doctor and a scan are the only ways to tell for sure what's going on and why.

Lifestyle in early pregnancy

Many women don't discover they are pregnant until quite a way through their first trimester, sometimes due to irregular periods, other times due to being so busy they forget they haven't had a period. The problem with finding out late is that sometimes it can cause lots of anxiety about the way you have been living. Which is why it cannot be said enough that unknowingly living a normal life as a non-pregnant person when you're actually in the early stages of pregnancy will not cause irreparable damage to your baby. What's important is not the time you fell over drunk, smoked a cigarette and stayed up all night, but what you do from now on to ensure your pregnancy is healthy.

"I used to party like a crazy person. In fact, the worst time I ever got drunk was when I was actually eight weeks pregnant and didn't know it. When I found out I cried for days thinking I'd damaged my baby, but she came out just fine."

Lauren, 28

Help! I've lost my mind (how being pregnant really makes you feel)

Joy, euphoria, happiness and bliss are the usual guaranteed feelings when you find out you're pregnant, but as strong as these feelings are, you'll soon find other emotional elements entering the scene and turning you from your usual normal self into someone you perhaps don't quite know. Here are the emotional changes your midwife or doctor won't warn you about:

Forgetfulness

Early pregnancy and forgetfulness do tend to go hand in hand. If you're not stumbling over words, you'll probably forget your ATM pin number, car keys or even your surname. It's a very common part of pregnancy, firstly because, let's face it, you now have a lot on your mind, and secondly because the energy that usually feeds your memory and your brain is being diverted away by your little darling to help him or her grow and develop. Because much of the baby's essential development goes on in the first trimester (first 12 weeks) you'll find that this is when your forgetfulness will be at its worst. It's not a medical problem, so don't worry and, contrary to popular opinion that brain function diminishes during pregnancy, news studies show that pregnant women's brains actually work better during pregnancy to cope with all the challenges the body is under.

Constant PMS

Do your moods change faster than the weather? Do you find yourself constantly weeping at adverts and losing your sense of humour with friends and family? Does it feel a bit like constant PMS? If so, you're not imagining it, you're just pregnant. Many, many women associate the feelings of early pregnancy with having a bad dose of PMS, mostly due to the early pregnancy hormone surge that mimics the symptoms of PMS: mood swings, irrational anger, tiredness and bloating. It will pass as you move out of the first trimester.

Lack of concentration

Are you feeling mentally fuzzy and unable to concentrate, especially at work? A preoccupation with being pregnant is partially the cause, as are hormonal changes (again) that affect your cognitive function (that's your ability to do everyday things like work, drive and pay attention). If everything, including work projects, paying bills, and appointments and meetings, seem to slip by, you need to rest more (tiredness makes this symptom worse) and give yourself ample reminders of what you need to do.

Anxiety about motherhood

Every single pregnant woman worries she's not up to the job of motherhood (just ask your own mum), and it's a worry that constantly nags away throughout pregnancy. If you're a high-flying kind of career girl, with an over-achieving perfectionist streak, it's likely to worry you even more, because that's part of your personality profile. What you have to realise is that lesser people than you bring up babies very well every day, and motherhood and pregnancy is not an exam you'll be marked on.

Fears about having regrets

Worrying that you'll regret having a child is a very common anxiety. It's partly fuelled by the fact that you know your life is changing in a huge way and partly by the fact that you're on a one-way street and you can't turn back. What you have to remind yourself is that you want this baby more than you don't want it and that you haven't yet factored your baby into your life: that's who the baby will be and how you'll love him or her and their personality.

Insanity

Irrational behaviour is also very common in the early days of pregnancy (ask the partners of your pregnant friends). Maybe your usual calm and sorted self will become an angry harridan who loses her temper all the time or cries at the drop of a hat. Or maybe, as one woman recently said, 'You will sit at the computer and realise you have forgotten how to use it.' Insanity is a by-product of pregnancy, especially in the first trimester, and it stems from the fact that you have a lot on your mind. Take it easy, relax, ease your busy schedule and normal service will resume before you know it.

tip

The more you talk about your fears the better and less stressed you will feel.

Morning sickness

The most nauseating fact about morning sickness and the thing you will hear the most – usually when you're stuck over a toilet bowl or desperately trying not to gag – is that it is a completely normal part of pregnancy and is a symptom that up to 75 per cent of women experience. 'Poor you', someone will say and then attempt to give you the best cure or solution. And your response will be to want to hit them, which you could blame on hormones or the fact that when you are constantly vomiting and nauseated, nothing is helpful.

There is no known cure for morning sickness, and you may find that what helps one person won't help you. Your doctor is likely to advise you to rest, eat regularly (small snacks and meals, and often) and see it as a good sign that all is going well. Below are a selection of lazy girl mum tips that are also worth trying out.

What to eat:
Kerry, 30, found that 'eating small bowls of cereal instead of full meals kept my sickness at bay. I think it was the fact that I didn't have to cook and the cereal was so bland that it helped. Also it kept my blood sugar level so helped ease the nausea.'

What to avoid:
Lynne, 27, found it best to avoid 'anything too heavy, too rich, spicy or flavoured. I found dried fruit and nuts good, and plain toast'.

"Don't overdo it. Getting tired and forgetting to eat were key factors in making my morning sickness worse."

Maria, 35

What to try:
Lara, 32, 'used my daughter's travel sickness acupressure bands and they really helped keep the nausea away, plus they are cheap and easy to use.' And Cam, 27, found that 'Ginger

is a lifesaver with morning sickness. Try ginger snaps, crystallised ginger pieces (from health shops), and ginger tea. It worked all three times for me.'

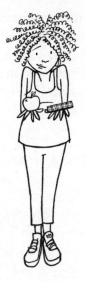

The good news

It might be hard to believe that morning sickness is good news, but generally doctors and midwives believe it is a good thing (see box for when it's not): you're being flooded with sickness because your body is being flooded with pregnancy hormones, which is good for the baby and a sign that your pregnancy is going in the right direction. Better still, despite your fears, morning sickness won't harm your baby, partly because the baby is like a parasite in your body stealing all the good nutrients and energy it needs from you. So, while you feel terrible, the baby will be doing just fine. What's more, researchers at the Hospital for Sick Children in Toronto now believe it could also be linked to the developing baby's brain. They conducted a five-year study to look at the long-term effects of morning sickness on the brains of babies and found that children whose mothers suffered from morning sickness during pregnancy were more likely to have higher IQ scores than those whose mothers had no symptoms.

If you're keen to try an alternative therapy, give acupuncture a go. Research shows that it's extremely effective in treating morning sickness, with one study showing that even after one treatment, symptoms can be reduced.

Extreme morning sickness

Known as hyperemesis gravidarum (HG), extreme morning sickness affects about 1 per cent of pregnant women. Symptoms are persistent nausea and vomiting (sometimes 20 to 30 times a day). As a result, a woman will lose between 10 and 20 per cent of her body weight, and become dehydrated, which is why women suffering from HG are admitted to hospital for intravenous hydration to stop liver damage.

Most women experience morning sickness from about six weeks of pregnancy and it lasts until 12–16 weeks, when pregnancy hormones start to balance out; however, some women do suffer for longer or find that the nausea and vomiting returns in the last trimester.

20 *ways*
to stay calm when pregnant

1 Try an alternative therapy
Many women find that alternative therapies, such as reflexology and pregnancy massage, help them get through the first trimester and not only deal with the morning sickness phase but also anxiety and stress.

2 Go to bed early
In the first trimester you need about ten hours of sleep a night, so that means going to bed earlier, cutting down on your social life and relaxing when you're at home.

3 Don't worry about what lies ahead
Anecdotal stories about terrible labours, miscarriages and morning sickness won't help alleviate your own fears. Remember, for every bad story there is a good one.

4 Seek help from trusted sources only
That's doctors you know, books that have been recommended and Internet sites that are well known or attached to a medical facility.

5 Talk to your partner
Don't assume he knows how you're feeling, or assume you know how he's feeling. Different people respond to pregnancy news in different ways.

6 Listen to the latest advice

Your mum may have had four children, but it's been a long time since she was pregnant. So, as helpful as she wants to be, don't take her advice if it feels wrong. If in doubt ask your midwife.

7 Accept that your life is changing

Many people say they aren't going to let pregnancy change them and that they intend to carry on as before. This is bad news for your energy and emotional levels. A pregnancy is a life-changing event (and that doesn't have to be a bad thing) but denying it's going to have an impact is a recipe for disaster.

8 Get informed on the medical stuff

Pregnancy is scary and frightening, not to mention confusing, which is why your best bet is to become informed so that you understand what's happening month by month and the risks associated with your choices as your pregnancy advances (see Resources for the best pregnancy websites).

9 Don't make any big life decisions

Who knows what you'll do when the baby comes. Don't make your life more stressful now by making any big decisions before you have to, about work, childcare, labour and breastfeeding issues.

10 Know your medical history

If possible, find out all you can about your parents' and your in-laws' medical histories before your first booking appointment with your midwife/GP. This is to rule out genetic illnesses that may affect your pregnancy and baby.

11 Don't go on a spending spree

There is plenty of time to buy baby stuff, and you don't have to get everything sorted by 12 weeks (remember, you have 40 weeks to get through). Plus, if you're worried about money, think about what you can borrow. Plenty of mums have clothes, equipment and toys they'll be only too pleased to pass on.

12 Relieve your stress with exercise

That's prenatal exercise, such as swimming and regular walking. Prenatal yoga and Pilates are also good, although you can't do these until the second trimester.

13 Wear loose clothing

Although you won't be showing yet, you may feel your clothes getting tighter and more restrictive. Instead of feeling as if you're about to 'pop out', wear looser clothes until you feel you can make the move to maternity wear.

14 Don't stress about your changing body

Thanks to the celebrities that go through pregnancy stick thin and then swing back to a size 8 five minutes after giving birth, it's easy to assume that weight gain during pregnancy is bad, when in fact it's essential for pregnancy. Remember that now is not the time to freak out about your body (for more on this see Chapter 3).

15 Don't stress about what you're eating

Worrying that you're eating all the wrong things or fattening foods you usually avoid is another way to get super-stressed. Relax. If you're feeling ill, eat what you can, and in the second trimester when you feel better focus on healthier foods.

16 Try not to make your whole life about being pregnant

You're pregnant, not ill, so you don't have to make your whole life about being pregnant (even if you want to). For starters it will bore everyone around you and secondly, you'll lose sight of the bigger picture, which is you're in a transition phase and soon your whole life is going to be about babies and children.

17 Take it easy

At the same time you don't have to be superwoman and try to prove to everyone that despite your pregnancy you can still do everything, such as working a 60-hour week, going to the gym daily and partying like an animal.

18 Make your commute easier

Commuting to work is stressful even when you're not pregnant, so help yourself by asking your employer if you can change your work hours to avoid rush hour, particularly if you use public transport. Make sure you always sit down while travelling, and if you are not offered a seat you should ask for one. Don't feel embarrassed – 99 per cent of people are only too willing to give up their seat for a pregnant woman.

19 Pamper yourself regularly

Beauty treatments, pregnancy massages, lush maternity body creams, these are all perfect ways to make yourself feel good during pregnancy, as well as relieving stress and anxiety at the end of a tiring day.

20 Laugh about it

Pregnancy is hard on the body and mind, and sometimes when things feel awful you just have to laugh about it and remind yourself that it will be over before you know it and well worth it in the end.

CHAPTER TWO

Life, work, friends and pregnancy

There are a variety of ways to approach being pregnant. For most of us it's a mixture of the following. Firstly there is

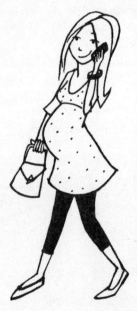

the Mumzilla road to motherhood, which involves trying to absorb every little detail there is to know about being pregnant, giving birth and having a baby. Then there is the I'm-just-going-to-wing-it technique, which means not picking up a single book and assuming that just because people have been having babies in fields for eons it will all be second nature. And finally there's the a-baby-will-just-have-to-fit-in-with-my-life method, which involves pretending pregnancy won't change your life at all and you can go on just as you are.

"I was one of those women who swore I was never going to let pregnancy turn me into a 'mummy-type', so for the first five months I carried on as usual. Then I was diagnosed with stress-related hypertension, which my doctor said indicated that I was doing too much. He pointed out that as much as I wanted to be the same person, I wasn't and needed to take into account the baby's health as well as mine."

Ally, 34

Of course, these are all radical ways of dealing with being pregnant, and most women fall between a few of these approaches. What you need to know if you're in the throes of working out how to handle being pregnant is that research shows that when you're pregnant what pays is to walk a middle path; that is, don't let being pregnant take over your life, but at the same time don't pretend it isn't going to affect your life.

The good news is you don't have to read everything and do everything the books/leaflets/midwives say when you're pregnant, especially if you're keen to carry on as normal for as long as possible; however, it does pay to be informed. So, be informed about what being pregnant means for you, your life and your new baby.

Know the basics

At the barest minimum, what you should know is the following:

- When your baby is due.
- What worrying pregnancy signs to look out for.
- Who to call if you're worried.
- What lifestyle changes to make and why.
- What pregnancy screening tests are and why you need them.
- What you're entitled too (depending on where you live, you will be entitled to everything from free dental care to a pregnancy grant).
- What happens in labour.
- What you can and can't do while pregnant.

Why bother? Well, because whether you feel physically fine or not, pregnancy is a condition that will affect your life and the people around you. This doesn't mean it will rock your life to its core, change your personality and forever put you in 'mummy-mode' but it does mean that on some level you have to accept that things are a-changing.

Physically, this means that your body is going to change whether you like it or not, so get to know what changes to expect and understand them for your own peace of mind and sanity (see Chapter 3 for more on this).

Being pregnant will change how people respond to you in your private life, social life and work life. This is because we all have our own agendas, so when someone we know says she is pregnant (be it a friend, family member or work colleague) we have a subjective response to it, whether it is happiness, boredom, jealousy, excitement or regret.

Understanding what makes the people you know tick when it comes to pregnancy can help stop you feeling crushed by an indifferent response or freaked out by an over-zealous one.

How being pregnant affects your friendships

Women, on the whole, are always happy to hear that their friends are pregnant, seeing it as ample opportunity to go for a shop at Baby Gap, enthuse about baby names and eventually calm their own biological clocks by playing with a small cute baby that they can give back when it starts screaming. This is why being pregnant can make friendships closer, as many women will tell you, and show you who your true friends are and help you to appreciate the women you know.

tip

Your friends will enjoy your pregnancy more if you don't make every conversation and meeting about your pregnancy.

However, like all things there will always be someone who isn't so happy for you. Usually the result of their own personal issues, and these so-called friends can blight a happy pregnancy, so here's how to deal with the friends that don't treat your news so positively.

Friends with issues

Those friends who have their own issues about pregnancy, such as infertility, being single and/or being too old for a baby, or sometimes a hidden issue that you won't ever know about, won't be happy to hear your news. If they are good friends they'll fake the joy and then keep away from you or admit they are envious and cry, while you dig deep for something sympathetic to say.

"Angie and I were such good friends until I got pregnant. Then she just stopped calling me. When I did see her she tried to pretend I was imagining that she had hardly ever contacted me, but I knew I wasn't. Sure enough, when Jake was born, she didn't even call. Mutual friends say she can't handle the fact I am married and have a child when she's still single."

Helen, 30

The key with these friends is to be understanding but not apologetic about your pregnant state. By being pregnant you haven't taken away their chance of getting pregnant, but only reminded them of what they haven't got. What's more, seeing someone pregnant when you can't have kids or have suffered a miscarriage, can be painful and devastating, hence friends who drop off your radar. There is not much you can do to stop them feeling this way, but what's important to realise is that it pays to pull back on your pregnancy enthusiasm when they are around and save the joyous stuff for the friends who want to hear it. Help yourself by:

- Giving them space to come to terms with your news.
- Not forcing an emotional confrontation; it won't end well.
- Assuming that if the tables were turned you wouldn't act like this (you may not, but who really knows).

Friends who are indifferent

Being pregnant and having babies is not everyone's idea of amazing news and an interesting event. Again, most good friends who aren't keen on having sprogs of their own are quite happy to hear that you're pregnant, but in the long term will be pretty indifferent to the highs and lows of you actually being pregnant. So, don't be crushed if they look bored when you show them a picture of your latest scan or roll their eyes when you talk about pushchairs and cribs.

"My best friend is so indifferent to my pregnancy it hurts. We went shopping for nursery furniture at the weekend and she spent the whole time yawning or sitting in a chair texting friends."

Anna, 28

Being bored about your pregnancy isn't a sign that they are not interested in you, but more that they don't need to hear everything there is to know about your pregnancy. A friendship has to be two ways to survive; that is, what about their life and what's happening to them? If you've stopped asking, don't be surprised when their eyes glaze over at the mere mention of the word 'pregnancy'. Help yourself by:

- Not taking it too personally. Remember, there are a hundred other people interested in your pregnancy besides them.
- Making your friendship about more than just your pregnancy.
- Keeping the nitty-gritty details of your pregnancy to friends who are keen to know.

Friends who are angry that they are 'losing' you

Being pregnant often means the days of endless shopping expeditions, drinking and partying and late-night chats on the phone are a thing of the past. This in itself can cause a lot of friction, especially if you're the first friend in your group to become pregnant or that being pregnant radically changes a friendship that is based on all of the above.

"One of my friends acts like my pregnancy is a personal attack on her. She suggested a weekend away in New York for her thirtieth and when I said I couldn't as I was due around that time she practically accused me of ruining her birthday on purpose and now won't speak to me."

Lizzie, 29

Although, logically, its ridiculous to be jealous of a baby bump, some friends can find the idea that you are no longer the old you quite threatening. The fear of losing a friend can also cause a person to act in ridiculous ways. Perhaps your friend will accuse you of no longer being interested in her, or of sidelining her in favour of your pregnant friends or even of having lied to her about your true self all these years.

There is not a lot you can do with friends like these except to keep reassuring them that you're still friends, albeit with different ideas of what it means to have fun. Help yourself by:

- Not trying to live up to their expectations.
- Reminding them that your friendship is based on more than going out and having a good time.
- Making time for them to do non-baby/pregnancy things.

Competitive pregnant friends

Being pregnant also does weird things to certain mums and pregnant friends. It can make a sane and relatively normal woman suddenly become pushy and horribly competitive, something which you may not have noticed when you were classed in the non-pregnant section of her address book.

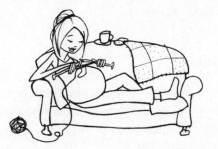

"I thought it would be wonderful to be pregnant at the same time as Lisa, but it isn't. She's always pointing out how 'large' my bump is compared to her 'neat' one and when I say I haven't yet done X or Y, she says, 'Really we did that ages ago'. She's really getting on my nerves."

Lena, 33

Dealing with competitive pregnant friends is a precursor to dealing with competitive mums, and if you play your cards right it can be fairly amusing. Firstly, do not let them pull you into their game. It can't be a competition if only one person is playing, so who cares if she can still wear her size 10 jeans and doesn't have to buy maternity? And who cares that her bump is already enrolled at nursery/university? Laugh her challenges off; she's the one feeling inadequate, which is why she's constantly trying to get one over you. Help yourself by:

- Telling her as little as possible about your pregnancy and plans.
- Laughing off her more childish attempts to rile you.
- Keeping your distance if her constant belittling is playing havoc with your hormones.

New Friends

Your new friends are the mum-to-be friends that you start to make when you get pregnant. Perhaps you'll meet them at the hospital, be introduced by other friends or meet at a childbirth class of some sort. Although you may think you don't need any more friends, becoming friends with women in the same position as you works well because you have a common link and someone who totally understands what you're going through not just when you're pregnant, but post labour and when you're struggling with a new baby. Best of all, new mum friends, once you have kids, can be a lifeline not only for sharing tips but also for babysitting and being an ideal play date with your baby.

"I met two wonderful new friends at a breastfeeding group. At the time I kept thinking they so weren't the usual kind of women I'd become friends with but they've proven to be worth their weight in gold. They were there at 2.00 a.m. when my child was sick and we have one night out a month where we just scream with laughter. Yes, they started off as mum friends but now they are definitely more than that."

Jo, 32

Help yourself to make mum friends by:

- Signing on for new parenting classes (this is the ideal spot to meet women who are pregnant and who live near you).
- Initiating friendships with pregnant women you think you'll get on with.
- Not making your friendship just about being pregnant.

5 ways to keep your friendships while pregnant

1. Remember, pregnancy is like an exotic holiday, only 100 per cent interesting if you've been there or are thinking of making the trip.
2. You may be feeling consumed by your pregnancy, but your friends lives are carrying on as normal, so make sure you listen as much as you speak.
3. Share your pregnancy as much as you can by asking your very best friends to be back up birth partners, godmothers or even helping you to arrange a baby shower.
4. Be honest about how you're feeling. Don't think you have to pretend to be happy about the pregnancy all the time.
5. Make time to do things you used to do (within reason); after all, you're pregnant for only nine months, then you'll really need your non-pregnant friends again for sanity, post-baby.

How being pregnant affects your working life

If you're like the majority of women, the chances are you are pregnant and working, and not just working but holding down a busy job that doesn't give you any leeway for being pregnant. The good news is that the first trimester is the hardest one as far as work is concerned, because it's the time when you feel the most vulnerable, tearful and ill, but after that being pregnant while working improves dramatically.

If you are lucky enough to have a sympathetic boss, you may have told him or her already and been given some slack, but if you're waiting to announce your news or are stuck with a by-the-book manager the chances are you're struggling to get through each day. Luckily, there are ways to make pregnancy and your working life easier. For starters, make sure that outside of work your time is spent relaxing and resting as much as possible. A crazy social life, and a busy work life do not make happy bedfellows during pregnancy!

Secondly, make sure you eat well at work. Skip the constant coffee drinking and sugary or fatty snacking side of office life and give yourself more energy to cope. Nutrition experts suggest keeping healthy snacks in your desk/bag (think oat cakes, dried fruit, bananas etc.), drinking eight glasses of water a day (dehydration being a massive side effect of being pregnant, which then makes fatigue worse) and taking regular breaks.

Thirdly, don't overdo it at work just to prove you can cope. In most countries there are strict regulations around pregnancy and work that mean you are protected against unfair treatment and have to be given time off for medical appointments. This means that once you tell your boss you are pregnant, your job should be given a risk assessment that ensures you don't have to:

- Lift or carry heavy loads
- Stand or sit for long periods
- Work long working hours

And that you aren't exposed to toxic substances.

If you feel you are being treated unfairly, or that you're being forced out of your job, seek advice and help (see Resources). In the meantime, here's how to cope:

Coping with co-workers

Co-workers can be tricky when it comes to pregnancy. Not only can they be gossipy about your condition or too forward about asking you questions about your pregnancy but they can also be ruthless about trying to get your job. Part of the problem is that being a co-worker is a weird halfway state between being friends and being strangers. People often think they know you more than they do, based on the fact that they see you constantly. What you have to do is draw firm boundaries about what you feel is acceptable co-worker behaviour and what isn't.

"One woman I work with kept coming up and rubbing my belly and commenting on how big I was. It really annoyed me, as previously the most we'd ever said was 'hello' to each other."

Leanne, 30

Mostly, navigating office politics when pregnant means keeping your pregnancy more to yourself than sharing all with the office and being sure not to let on what's affecting you and what isn't. With co-workers, the less they know, the less they can be offensive/overly helpful or nosy about. As for the ruder questions such as, 'Was it planned?' 'Boy you're SO big' and 'I didn't have you down as the mothering type', just say, 'That's very rude', and you'll be amazed at how quickly they back off. Help yourself by:

- Only discussing your pregnancy privately with certain work friends whom you know you can trust.
- Be clear about touching-the-bump boundaries; tell people your bump is off limits, as it's painful.

tip

> Don't feel you have to answer questions about maternity leave and returning to work with even your boss until you're ready. It's usually post-birth near to the end of your maternity leave when you'll have to make a definite decision.

Morning sickness at work - how to cope

Morning sickness and work definitely don't go hand in hand, but there are ways to help make it manageable. Firstly, being aware of what makes your morning sickness worse can help you learn to cope with it. For instance, is it worse when you haven't eaten or when you can smell food, or when you are tired or get too hot?

"My morning sickness was always worse by 4.00 p.m. when I'd be in the ladies literally over a sink. In the end my manager suggested I work from 8.00 till 4.00 p.m., rather than 9.00 till 5.00 p.m. and it's really helped. Leaving home at 7.00 a.m. is painful but it's always worth it at the end of the day."

Sam, 32

All these things happen at work and are easily alleviated. Firstly, make sure you eat every three hours, even if it's just a cracker or dry cereal. Secondly, go out of the office at lunchtimes so that you don't have to smell other people's lunches. Thirdly, change your work hours so you don't have to commute in the rush hour (standing up in a hot, crowded bus or train is a recipe for throwing up) and lastly, schedule meetings during the time of day when you feel best. If all these strategies fail, try to attack your morning sickness from another angle, such as alternative therapies or home remedies (see Chapter 1 for more on this). Help yourself by:

- Being honest about what's making your sickness worse in the office, such as smelly food or lack of air and ask to move to another desk.
- Asking your boss if you can change your work hours so that you can work around your worst times.

tip

Now is not the time to be super-employee and overdo the overtime. Tiredness exacerbates morning sickness.

Lack of concentration at work

Feeling devoid of work energy and the ability to concentrate is tough at work, especially if you have a job that demands your full attention or isn't at a desk and involves people directly working with you. Zero concentration skills are a by-product of the first trimester and, hopefully, by weeks

14–16 you'll have rediscovered your zest for hard work. In the meantime here's how to combat it.

Firstly, it's easy to let lack of concentration turn into wasted days and weeks, and eventual work panic, so come up with a daily plan to get at least three things done a day. Knowing what daily targets you have to hit can help remind you of where your focus should be. Next, try to pinpoint what's behind your lack of attentiveness: are you distracted by being pregnant and too busy surfing pregnancy sites? If so, limit your browsing to lunch hours. Is fatigue the enemy? If so, get important and vital work done in the mornings before the day wears you down.

Do you feel trapped in a persistent fog? You're not alone; pregnancy can make you feel like this. The way out is to make yourself focus on one important element and take a step-by-step approach to your job. One hour at a time, one day at a time. Help yourself by:

- Taking a few days off to recuperate, and coming back in with a plan.
- Asking for help from your line manager, if you're really struggling.

tip

If you really can't cope with the sickness and tiredness and you feel ill, see your doctor for a sick note.

Your view of your job, salary and finances

Where once you would happily spend half your salary on a holiday/bag/outfit, there is nothing like being pregnant to make you wish you hadn't taken quite so many taxis or bought so many pair of shoes over a lifetime. If finances and your salary (or lack of it) are on your mind, you're not alone. Not only is the media fond of telling us all just how much a child costs over a lifetime but you're probably also worrying about how you're going to afford to be a working mum.

The bad news is that being pregnant is a very bad time to look for a new job or a promotion and/or to start working for yourself. Not only will you lose money via your maternity package if you leave but also, even though employers aren't allowed to discriminate against pregnant women, very few are likely to give a job to a woman who's about to take 9–12 months off.

The good part about staying where you are is that you may be able to negotiate better working hours post-maternity leave, because your employer knows your worth (in most countries your employer has to at least entertain the idea) and you may have landed yourself a spectacular maternity package in the meantime (see the human resources department in your company for more on this). Whatever your deal, sit tight and don't jack in your job, or make mutterings that you may not be back – well, not until you know for sure what it is you want to do post-baby (for more on money and baby worries see Chapter 5).

5 Tips to keep your boss happy while you're pregnant

1. Don't rely on colleagues to pick up your slack; it won't endear you to them or your boss.
2. Be honest about how you're coping. He or she will have their suspicions anyway.
3. Ask for time off or help when you need it, not when you can't be bothered to work.
4. Be aware that it's in your interests to keep your boss happy, especially if you're seeking a change in your working hours post-baby.
5. Don't overcompensate by working harder; it will only backfire on your health. You're only pregnant for nine months.

How being pregnant affects your relationship

Has your husband/boyfriend dropped from his demi-god status to most annoying man in history in just a few weeks? Does everything he says drive you to distraction, annoy you or just remind you that he has no idea what you're going through? If so, you're not alone. There's nothing like pregnancy to make you realise that the man you love can also be the man who drives you crazy.

However, there is also nothing like a pregnancy to make you act and think irrationally, behave badly and overreact to every innocent comment thrown your way. In many ways you have to pity the poor guy. Yes, he doesn't know what it's like to be pregnant, but that's not his fault and, let's be honest, you don't know what it's like to live, eat and sleep with a pregnant woman?

If your relationship is currently in the 'honeymoon' stage of your pregnancy, you're probably swearing that the above is never going to happen to you and that you will never scream, 'You DON'T understand!' 'Why aren't you LISTENING?' and 'I HATE YOU!', during your pregnancy, and all power to you if you achieve this; however, bear in mind that no matter how secure, strong and loving your relationship is, being pregnant will affect it at some level. It might be by having a partner who is too involved, not involved enough or has wildly different views to you.

---

5 Annoying partner comments

1. 'You're overreacting.'
2. 'You used to be more fun before you were pregnant.'
3. 'Should you be eating that?'
4. 'Of course, you look fat, you're pregnant.'
5. 'Oh my God! Are you being sick again?'

I hate my partner!

Of course, there are rational reasons to hate your partner when you're pregnant. Perhaps he's run off with his PA, told you he's gay or that you're officially bankrupt. Then there are the irrational reasons such as: you're feeling so ill you're blaming him for everything; he's not making you feel better; he's not giving you enough attention; and/or he's disinterested in every small nuance of being pregnant. Or perhaps he's just being annoying and inconsiderate. Whichever it is, the list of what irks when you're pregnant is endless.

"My biggest bugbear is the constant stupid joking my boyfriend makes whether we're at the doctor's, at home or when I am throwing up. He thinks it distracts me, but it makes me want to kill him."

Isabella, 30

What you have to remember is that being pregnant is a steep learning curve for both of you. After all, this may be his first time through pregnancy as well, and although he can't possibly understand what it feels like for you, it's unlikely you can understand the anxiety of having a pregnant partner who is unwell and unhappy and scared. Part of the problem is that when we feel anxious and unwell we look to our partner to make us feel better, but at the same time we feel annoyed when they dare to make suggestions and angry when they throw their hands up in despair. If you want to avoid the I-hate-you route, then you need to tell your partner what it is you need him to do, whether that's to listen more often, tell you it's going to be OK or simply be more attentive. Help yourself by:

- Trying to understand where he's coming from. He can't feel what you feel, so it's a bit of a non-event at the moment, which doesn't mean he's not interested.

- Buying him a book that's designed for new fathers and pregnancy so that he can see he's not alone.
- Not expecting him to second-guess your every desire and need.

No sex/too much sex

With a normal pregnancy (that is, a pregnancy with no complications), you can keep having sex right up until labour starts. This is because sex is not linked with miscarriage or harm to the baby. As for fears about infection and the baby getting squished, rest assured that a plug seals your cervix, so infection can't get through, and the muscles of the uterus protect your baby from getting hurt.

fact

A baby will squirm and move about after sex and orgasm but not because he/she felt it but because your heart rate has speeded up.

The problem with sex during pregnancy is differing sex drives: either you want it and he doesn't, or your partner doesn't because he has fears about sex during pregnancy. Many men feel 'weird' about having sex with a baby sitting in your tummy, especially if the baby starts kicking wildly in the midst of your passion. If this is the case, reassure your partner that the baby (1) doesn't know what's going on; (2) can't feel it; and (3) is kicking because your heart rate has increased.

"My husband is freaked out by having sex when I am pregnant. It's almost like I have become a sacred vessel that can't be touched."

Gill, 28

If your partner treats you as if you are made of porcelain and can't be touched, consider two things. One, how are you behaving? Are you leading him to believe that you are delicate and in need of special care? In which case this is likely to work against your sexual image. Two, does he have certain beliefs about pregnant women being fragile? In which case you need to dispel those for him. Remind him that pregnancy isn't an illness and that you are still the woman he's known all these years.

If you haven't been in the mood since getting pregnant, you're also not alone. Hormones directly affect the libido and self-esteem, which means that if you're feeling self-conscious about your bigger body, or a bit low in general, you won't feel like having sex. Usually this happens in the first and third trimester, so your sex life will pick up in weeks 12–27.

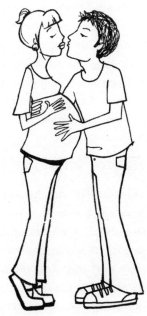

On the other hand you may feel 'mad for it' and desperate for sex all the time. Again, this is down to your hormones, and if your partner's willing, go for it. If he's not, or your desire is a massive deviation from your usual sex drive, try to compromise and indulge in other types of sexual play besides full-on intercourse every time.

Finally, don't be worried that you won't enjoy sex with your new and ever-changing body, studies show sex is even better for some women during pregnancy, as increased blood flow to the pelvic area can heighten sensation and orgasm. If you're not one of those women, don't despair, your sex drive and your ability to enjoy sex will come back once the baby is born, so hang on in there. Help yourself by:

- Remembering that even if you don't feel like having sex, being intimate in any way is good for your relationship, especially during pregnancy.
- As your pregnancy progresses, you may find that the missionary position (man on top) is not comfortable any more. Try lying partly sideways, which allows your partner to keep most of his weight off your uterus.
- Experiment with positions on a regular basis, because the more your bump grows the more experimental you may have to become.

He's too interested in your pregnancy

Believe it or not, partners who are too interested in your pregnancy can be just as annoying as partners who aren't interested at all. Having someone eagerly point out all the details of your pregnancy, tell you what you're feeling and why, and why X is normal and you shouldn't moan about it, probably makes you want to scream. Aside from feeling suffocated, it's just irritating to contend with.

"My husband was so into the pregnancy that you'd have thought he was carrying our daughter. He'd email me 'interesting' facts about ten times a day, call me to tell me what to eat and grill the midwives and doctors at my appointments. I ended up feeling as if he was sucking the joy out of being pregnant."

Seema, 29

Partners who are over-interested in your pregnancy act like this simply because they want to feel connected to the growing baby and want to parent right from the word go. What they forget is that in doing so they've forgotten all about you and what you need and want. Try telling him that you need to discover some of the facts for yourself and, while it's great he's so involved, he's also crowding you and you need space. Perhaps designate areas he can be in charge of, such as labour information or what pushchair to buy, what car seat, or which hospital has the best care. Make him feel useful and you'll avoid an all out war. Help yourself by:

- Reminding yourself that his behaviour, although annoying, is normal, especially if he's someone who throws himself into projects heart and soul.
- Being kind. He thinks he's being supportive, so be kind when you tell him he's not.
- Finding ways for him to be involved that don't irritate you.

Differing views on parenting and pregnancy

There is nothing like having a child together to bring up the differing views we all hold about pregnancy and parenting. In many ways this is understandable, as we are all a product of our own backgrounds, whether we intend to parent just like our parents did or in a completely opposite way. The problem is that having very different views on pregnancy can drive a huge wedge between the two of you before the baby even arrives and cause long-lasting resentment.

"We disagree so much. Ian is a huge believer in natural home birth, with no painkillers, whereas I'd feel safer in a hospital with options. He thinks I should eat healthily and exercise during pregnancy, while I feel too tired and in need of comfort food. We argue and fight about every aspect of being pregnant."

Nina, 32

What you have to remember is that much of the way we think we will parent will be diluted and compromised once our child comes along, something we can't really fathom in the pregnancy stage; however, feeling as if a partner is policing your pregnancy because he has strong views about how you should do it is bad news, so don't let major decisions be decided for you without thinking about what you want and why. Ultimately, the baby is part of both of you, but the pregnancy is about your body and what you feel you can cope with, not what your partner feels you should do because he's read about it, or his mum did it that way. Help yourself by:

- Setting firm boundaries around your own health and issues, such as delivery, that allow you to ultimately have the final say.
- Asking your midwife or doctor for help, if you feel unable to do the above. Ultimately, they will always take your preference (as you are the patient) over your partner's.
- Telling your partner how he's making you feel.

---

5 Ways to keep your relationship happy

1. Don't make everything about being pregnant.
2. Ask your partner how he's feeling about being a new parent.
3. Talk about your backgrounds and how they have affected your view of parenting.
4. Ask friends who are parents for pointers on parenting and relationships.
5. Have some fun; once you have a new baby you'll be too tired to go out.

Pregnancy and your social life

What social life, you may be thinking? In between morning sickness, fatigue and not being able to drink you might be currently feeling that your social life is non-existent and a precursor to what you have to look forward to as a new mum. The good news is, despite what some mothers say, pregnancy and a new baby will not kill your social life, just alter it.

You don't want to party any more

For a start, what the grumpy mums don't say is that the change is often a welcome one. Not many pregnant women want to dance the night away in Jimmy Choo heels and survive on four hours sleep and a late-night kebab for dinner. Neither do they want to wake up with a hangover (and I'm not even talking about the health warnings over drink) or battle partying fatigue with pregnancy fatigue. When you get pregnant, the first thing you start to do, consciously or not, is to pare back your social life to what you feel you can cope with.

"I used to love clubbing till the early hours, but now that I crave my bed by 9.30 I just can't do it any more, so it was an easy decision to make."
Leanne, 26

That's not to say you won't miss your pre-pregnancy social life, because you will. It's likely you'll find yourself lusting after the latest new fashions, battling the desire to wear your sexiest and your highest heels, and feel swamped with envy when your girlfriends tell you what a fantastic and hedonistic time they are having without you. What you have to remember is that pregnancy is not a life sentence, it lasts nine months, and by this time next year you can do all of the above and more (with a bit of planning). Help yourself by:

- Suggesting alternative nights out such as a dinner at yours, or lunch at weekends.
- Don't be afraid to say no to going out, it's a temporary thing and won't ruin your life.
- Be realistic about what you can cope with and what you can't.

You feel too vulnerable to be out

Feeling vulnerable about your pregnant state is another one of those unspoken pregnancy things. For a start, it's very normal and very common to feel worried when you're out – after all your body has changed radically, you have something very special growing inside and you want to protect it as much as you can.

"When I was pregnant with my first daughter I was so ridiculous, I wouldn't pump petrol because I was afraid it would harm her."

Jackie, 34

If feeling vulnerable has become another reason why you may feel you can't socialise as normal, it's important to get your fears into perspective. Your baby is well protected inside your uterus and going out isn't putting baby in danger, even if you get jostled on public transport. If you still feel too vulnerable to go to your usual haunts, speak up and tell friends and your partner; sometimes airing your fears can make you feel better. If your anxiety becomes too much, or you start to feel you can't do everyday things, speak to your midwife and doctor, as they can help.

fact

About 10 per cent of women suffer from depression and anxiety during pregnancy.

Help yourself by:

- Socialising at weekends and during the day instead of at night.
- Practising moving slightly out of your comfort zone every day. It will help to increase your confidence.
- Writing down what's making you feel vulnerable and anxious, and see if you can face it head on.

Antenatal depression

Pregnancy is supposed to be a happy time, but it's also a time of stresses and anxieties, especially if you're worried about money, your job or you are having relationship problems. Studies show that an estimated 10 per cent of women struggle with antenatal depression during their pregnancy, which can then lead to postnatal depression if not treated. If you're feeling persistent sadness, lack of confidence, constant anxiety and even fear, you may have antenatal depression.

You must tell someone how you feel – a friend or a family member and your doctor and midwife. There is much they can do to help you feel better, reassured and less anxious so that you can get through your pregnancy.

Socialising - *what you can do*

You don't have to lie in bed for nine months making friends with the TV guide, because you can still socialise, party and have fun. The trick is to do it in moderation and during the right trimester. The first trimester is the worst time to try to pretend to have a social life, but sadly it is also the time when you'll want to pretend you can still have one.

Help yourself by choosing pregnancy-appropriate days and nights out: the movies, dinner and seeing friends, over clubbing, mad parties and endless shopping trips. Be smart about what you choose, for the sake of your health, because although you may feel fine while you're overdoing it, at some point your body will rebel. In the first trimester, especially, all your body's nutrients and energy are being diverted away from you into making your baby, so less is always more.

Remember, if you are having a normal pregnancy with no complications you can still do everything you used to do in your leisure time within reason, such as exercise, go swimming, dancing, hiking and running. Extreme sports are not recommended, for obvious reasons, but no one can stop you if that's what you really want to do.

Better still, change the record and schedule-in some girlie pamper days either at a local day spa or at home. Not only will they keep you close to your girlfriends but they will also help you to relax and enjoy your time with them.

What you can't do

You can't drink (in an OTT, binge-drinking way) smoke and take drugs – all things that you know you shouldn't do, because it's probably been drummed into your head a million times by your health-care provider, not to mention friends and perfect strangers.

You can't drink more than one unit a week (although this official figure will vary depending on which country you live in); for example, current UK guidance recommends that not drinking during pregnancy is the safest option; however, the issue is confusing as official advice also says that drinking up to four units a week is not harmful. If you are confused or worried about drinking, your midwife can offer advice. She can also help increase your awareness about the harmful effects of alcohol, especially if you have not been aware of the need to cut down. Advice is especially relevant during the first three months (first trimester) of pregnancy when your baby's major organs, including their brain, spinal cord and facial features, are developing.

Smoking, even socially (when you have about ten or less a day), while you're pregnant is also a big no-no! Countless scientific studies show that smoking is not only bad for your health but also that of your baby. Not only does the habit cause low birth-weight babies, who may be born with an increased risk of asthma, but smoking also increases your baby's risk of sudden infant death syndrome (SIDS). Statistics suggest that the risk of SIDS is four times higher if you smoke between one and nine cigarettes a day when pregnant, and eight times higher if you smoke 20 cigarettes a day or more. Smoking during pregnancy has also been linked to:

1. Poor health for you, with an increased chance of:
   - Miscarriage
   - Bleeding
   - Nausea and morning sickness
2. And poor health for your baby, such as:
   - Slow growth
   - Premature birth
   - Stillbirth

The problem is that when you smoke you inhale over 4,000 chemicals into your body. Two of the main components are tar and carbon monoxide, which then get into your bloodstream and cut down the amount of oxygen reaching your baby. Babies who don't get enough oxygen grow at a slower rate, so tend to be born smaller and weaker.

Stopping smoking will benefit your baby's health immediately as well as in the long term, because when your lungs become smoke-free, the carbon monoxide and chemicals clear from your body and your oxygen levels return to normal. This means that there's more oxygen in your blood, making you and your baby much healthier and lowering the risk of premature birth, miscarriage and the risk of SIDS.

International guidelines on drinking and pregnancy

One unit of alcohol is 8g, which equals half a pint of beer or cider or a small glass of wine.

Australia 10g of alcohol
Advice: maternal alcohol consumption can harm the developing foetus or breastfeeding baby.

Canada 13.6g of alcohol
Advice: although the prudent choice for women who are or may become pregnant is to abstain from alcohol, small amounts of alcohol occasionally during pregnancy shows that the risk to the foetus in most situations is likely to be minimal.

Ireland 10g of alcohol

Advice: stopping drinking during pregnancy is the safest advice. Baby's vital organs, for example, heart, brain and skeleton, are formed between 10–50 days after conception. Often, this is before you know you are pregnant. Cutting down or stopping alcohol while trying to become pregnant protects your baby.

Switzerland 10g of alcohol

Advice from the Swiss Institute for the Prevention of Alcohol and Drug Addiction: if you do decide to drink, do not drink more than one glass per day, and do not drink every day.

United Kingdom 8g of alcohol

Advice: pregnant women should not drink more than 1–2 units of alcohol once or twice a week and should not get drunk.

United States 14g of alcohol

Advice: pregnant women should avoid drinking alcohol.

20 ways
to stay sane when pregnant

1 Keep telling yourself that you're pregnant, not ill
Keep reminding yourself that you are carrying a baby, not in need of special care. Thinking you're more delicate than you are will stop you from living your life and enjoying your pregnancy.

2 Visualise the bigger picture
Remembering what this pregnancy is all about – that is, a new baby – can help you get through the tougher moments when you're feeling down, ill and tired.

3 Enjoy being pregnant
Revel in being pregnant and make the most of it, because it's over in just nine months and one day you'll look back and wish you'd taken more pleasure in it.

4 Stay in bed more often
You may or may not be able to get much sleep once the baby is born, so make the most of it now with naps, lie-ins and more time spent in bed. Doctors recommend sleeping on your side with your knees bent to increase blood flow. Try putting a small pillow under your bump and one between your knees to help support your back.

5 Don't worry about gaining weight

Everyone gains weight during pregnancy, because your body needs more food to grow a baby, support it and bring on the milk. So, relax about what you eat and forget the diet for once in your life.

6 Stop planning how to lose the baby weight

Contrary to what people say, the reality of baby weight is nine months on and nine months off. So don't go down the back-in-my-jeans-by-three-weeks route and you'll be much happier.

7 Don't let other people police your pregnancy habits

If you're being sensible and are making informed decisions, don't let loved ones and strangers start telling you what you should and shouldn't be doing. Pregnancy doesn't make you public property.

8 Give yourself a break

You don't have to be the perfect pregnant woman – pregnancy advice is there in abundance but that doesn't mean you have to follow it by the book. If you have no time to exercise, just walk about in your lunch hour. No time to make healthy home-cooked meals? Just ensure that you eat your five a day. No time to relax? Then go to bed earlier!

9 Take one day at a time

As in take one pregnancy day at a time. You don't need to freak yourself out about labour if you're only 12 weeks, and you don't need to worry about baby routines if you're in your second trimester, and you definitely don't need to worry about being a working mother when you've only just had your baby.

10 Ignore old wives' tales

They are amusing but that's all. Pregnancy old wives' tales are just that – tales – meaning, there is no scientifically proven basis for what they say, and they are just there to worry you or make you think you have to do something you don't. Ignore, ignore, ignore!

11 Make yourself relax

Aside from feeling better, allow yourself the chance to sit on the sofa and do nothing. While it's normal to feel guilty about this, it's also important to realise that once you have a baby this will be a thing of the past, so enjoy it now.

12 Research some relaxation techniques

Relaxation techniques will not only help to slow you down and bliss you out, but they will also benefit you during labour (see Resources for more on this).

13 Educate yourself about what's happening to you

Understanding the pregnancy process and what changes to look out for will alleviate your fears about being pregnant and help you to feel more in control.

14 Don't share your thoughts on baby names

… because some annoying person will tell you that it's a ridiculous/common/silly and/or weird name, and it will drive you crazy.

15 Do some exercise!

Even if it's just 30 minutes walking a day! Exercise not only lifts your mood, but it also helps your poor aching pregnant body deal with the extra load you're carrying.

16 Forget trying to make your baby smart

Eat more fish, play him Mozart, read to him, and teach him Einstein's theory of relativity or give the poor bump a break (and yourself). None of these things are proven, and are just a way to make you feel as if you should be hot-housing your child before he's even born.

17 Don't worry about postnatal depression

If you feel you're prone to it or that you may already be depressed, speak to your doctor and midwife as soon as possible. When it comes to depression and pregnancy, the sooner you seek help the better the outcome.

18 Look after your looks

Your skin, hair and nails all change significantly when you are pregnant. Sometimes for the better, and sometimes for the worse, which is why taking the time to take care of your looks pays off, not only in terms of maintenance but also in self-esteem.

19 Have some sex before you go to sleep

It will help you to feel closer to your partner, release some feel-good endorphins and help you to relax before bed.

20 Don't sweat the small stuff

There's nothing like pregnancy to make you worry about everything from space issues at home to how you're going to afford to bring up a child and be a good working mum. The answer is to take each day as it comes, face each issue as it arises and refuse to do more than that.

CHAPTER THREE

Pregnancy health

Whether you've been a true lazy girl prior to getting pregnant and done zero towards good health or simply put your health needs at the bottom of your busy to-do list, when you're pregnant it pays to prioritise your health. Not just for the sake of your baby but because you will feel truly awful if you don't get to grips with looking after your mind and body.

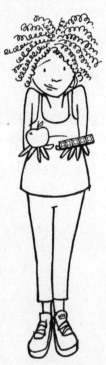

The good news is that pregnancy health is not rocket science, and while there is a host of medical stuff to get your head around (see Chapter 8 and your midwife) there is also a host of health stuff to consider and make decisions about. Of course, you can take the über-lazy route and ignore it all and do what you want, but bear in mind that the healthier your body is during pregnancy the better you will feel while being pregnant and the easier your labour will be.

Exercise: how and why you should get moving

When you talk to mums and pregnant women, there are many schools of thought on pregnancy and exercise. Some feel that exercising is a complete waste of time, especially if you're doing it to keep your weight down. On this front they are right. You will gain weight in pregnancy, so it's pointless trying to exercise in order to keep yourself in pre-pregnancy clothes.

Others feel you can't do much and it doesn't help anyway. On this point they are wrong. There is plenty you can do on the exercise front, and exercising throughout does plenty for your health and that of your baby.

fact

> Seventy-five per cent of pregnant women do no exercise!

Others feel it will endanger their pregnancy, which it may well do if you do very high-intensity exercise where you sweat buckets and nearly always pass out, or extreme sports where you put your life in danger, and/or try to keep going with your regular gym regime designed to suit you when you're not pregnant.

"I'm no great exerciser but I did find just going for a walk every day and going swimming every week helped me feel better during pregnancy."
Helen, 30

The reality is that moderate exercise is good for you during pregnancy. Not only is it associated with a better pregnancy outcome and a shorter labour but it will also improve your stamina for labour and help you to feel more in control of your body. Not that it means it will give you stronger uterine muscles to push the baby out (it won't), but more stamina means it will give you the strength to make it through your labour and deal with the exhaustion of the first stage of labour – your contractions – and the second stage of pushing. Being too exhausted to do these things increases your chances of having an assisted delivery or medical intervention.

Lastly, exercise will help strengthen your pelvic floor (the muscles that weaken during pregnancy and control your urge to pee), your posture and help you to relax. Ignore your pelvic floor muscles and there is a good chance you will be peeing your pants every time you sneeze, cough and laugh (it sounds scary, but it's true, ask any mum you know). Ignore looking after your posture and you're asking for nine months of backache as your bump gets bigger and pulls your body out of shape. Ignore learning to relax and you will have trouble sleeping and knowing how to relax during labour, which is vital if you want to recover between contractions.

These are some of the reasons to try to fit exercise into your already busy schedule. If that doesn't convince you, here are the myths versus the facts on pregnancy exercising.

Myth: never get your heart rate over 130 while exercising during pregnancy
There is no one heart rate that's right for every pregnant woman. You will know if your heart rate is too high because

you will feel sick and faint. Aim to work at a level where you feel slightly out of breath but can still talk normally.

Myth: it's not safe to do abdominal workouts during pregnancy
Although sit ups after the first trimester are a no-no, because you shouldn't be lying on your back, you also need to have a certain flexibility in your stomach muscles so that they can relax in between uterine contractions during labour (something that's difficult if you've been trying for a six-pack); however, abdominal work throughout your pregnancy – that is, while swimming and during Pilates and Yoga – is essential. It stops backache and helps to strengthen your pelvic floor.

Myth: you can't stretch during pregnancy or you'll injure yourself
During pregnancy, your body produces a hormone called relaxin that's designed to help lubricate your joints and make labour easier. This makes you more bendy during pregnancy, labour and the postnatal period, so you do have to be careful with deep muscle stretching, because you can go beyond what's good for your body; however, stretching is good during pregnancy, especially calf stretches and shallow squats, which help deal with the problems of water retention in the legs and maintain muscle for a range of positions during labour.

Myth: if you have never exercised before, now is not the time to start
Now is not the time to bring out your own miracle workout DVD, but now *is* the time to bring your activity levels up to help improve your fitness, your stamina and your energy levels.

Signs you need to stop exercising and seek medical advice

- Spotting and vaginal bleeding
- Fluid leaking from the vagina
- Decreased foetal movement
- Uterine contractions
- Calf swelling or pain
- Headache, and chest pain
- Shortness of breath
- Dizziness
- Feeling faint
- Joint swelling and problems
- Overheating

Essential pregnancy exercise

If you do just one thing when you're pregnant, make sure it's pelvic floor exercises. The pelvic floor is formed of layers of muscle (imagine a sling shape) that support the uterus, bowel, rectum and bladder. Usually, they work just fine, but pregnancy and childbirth put pressure on these muscles due to the weight of the baby, and as a result they weaken and you may find that you urinate slightly when you laugh, sneeze or cough, also known as 'stress incontinence'. It is also important to have good strength in the pelvic floor muscles because it will help you to push the baby out and stop you from being incontinent post-baby.

The greatest demand placed on these muscles is during labour and childbirth, as the pelvic floor stretches to its maximum to allow for the passage of the baby. This amount of stretching weakens the pelvic floor, which is why you need to do pelvic floor exercises during your pregnancy.

tip

Do your pelvic floor exercises whenever you can. Studies suggest that as many as 25 per cent of women experience incontinence post-baby.

The good news is that no matter how busy you are, you can tone these muscles so that they maintain their strength by doing regular 'invisible' exercises at your desk, in the car or even on the bus (although beware that in the beginning the exercises may make you want to pee).

All you have to do is:

1. Locate your pelvic floor muscles. These are the muscles you release when you are having a pee. To tense them, think upwards and back (so you're tensing from above the rectum and from above the vagina and have a sense of pulling upwards).
2. Hold for five seconds and then slowly relax.
3. Make sure you tense the muscles without holding your breath or pulling in your stomach muscles. The aim is to tense them, count to 5 and then slowly release to a count of 5 (the slow release is as important as the hold).
4. Aim to do ten sets of five exercises each day.

Great forms of pregnancy exercise

Walking The good news is you can do this from the beginning and build up from 10 minutes a day to 30 minutes.

Even better, the busiest person in the world can maintain a walking schedule by breaking up her exercise into three 10-minute chunks. So, get off the bus/tube one stop earlier, or park the car a bit further away, and walk to work. Walk at lunchtime, and walk on the way home.

Yoga You can't do Yoga until you are 14 weeks pregnant, but after that it's one of the best forms of gentle exercise. Not only will it help you to relax but it will also help to build stamina and strength.

Pilates Like Yoga, you can't do Pilates until you are 14 weeks pregnant, but after that it's an amazing exercise to improve posture, strengthen your stomach and back muscles (in a good way) and help you to feel in control of your pelvic floor.

Antenatal exercise classes Specialised antenatal exercise classes are based around all fitness levels and help give you an all-round workout – aerobic, anaerobic and stretching – that builds stamina and helps you to relax.

Swimming Pregnancy and swimming are ideal bed partners, simply because there is nothing like the buoyancy of water to take the stress off your joints and out of your body. It's relaxing, will keep you fit, is hard to overdo and is a pleasure all round.

What to be careful about

Running Even if you're a seasoned runner, be careful about overdoing the running. Apart from pressure on your joints due to the hormone relaxin, you need to make sure that you are wearing a well-fitted and comfortable sports bra so that your growing boobs don't end up with stretch marks from all the bouncing. Take it easy and work at a moderate level.

Lifting weights Now is not the time to build muscle, so do not lift heavy weights during pregnancy, especially above your head, because this runs the risk of tearing your placenta. Instead, go lighter and increase repetitions for muscle maintenance.

What to avoid

Contact sports Your centre of gravity has changed, which will make you more clumsy and increase your chances of injury, so avoid contact sports, although you can still do the exercises and workouts on a moderate level. Think shadow boxing, bag work and warm ups.

Extreme sports Remember, they are called 'extreme' for a reason, so why even risk it?

Food – what to eat and what not to eat

When it comes to food, nothing changes your appetite and sense of taste faster than being pregnant. You might be the healthiest woman in the world, but the second you get pregnant you could find yourself craving all kinds of stuff that you'd usually turn your nose up at.

"All I wanted was cheese sandwiches on nasty cheap white bread."

Hannah, 32

This is especially true in the first trimester when the body is busy diverting nutrients and energy away from you into making your baby. You could find that you're craving carbohydrates and fat, or feel so ill that all you can eat is crackers and cereal. Perhaps you'll gain a sweet tooth or crave something sour, or even want to eat coal (more common than you may think).

Although it's important to eat healthily if you're suffering from morning sickness, don't make your diet another thing to stress about. What's important at this stage is not what you eat, but to eat regularly and to eat something.

tip

Seventy-five per cent of women indulge food cravings during pregnancy while only 8 per cent reach for healthy substitutes. Think ahead and plan your snacks to combat this.

The second trimester, when your hormones settle down, is the time to focus on healthy and nutritious eating. Your body may be craving ice cream and chocolate or pizza every night but try to fight the urge, firstly because you'll feel better, secondly because it will be better for your baby, and thirdly because you'll gain less weight.

To avoid weight-related pregnancy problems, a nutrient-rich diet is key. Eat plenty of fruit and vegetables, protein, fibre, dairy and carbohydrates, and limit foods high in fat and sugar. This will not only help your baby to grow but it will also ensure that your weight rises in a steady way that won't leave you feeling depressed and concerned at a time when you should be feeling relaxed and happy about what's to come.

What to eat:

- **Fruit and vegetables** Aim for at least five portions of a variety each day.
- **Bread, pasta, rice and potatoes** Your body needs carbohydrates to help your baby develop.
- **Protein** such as lean meat and chicken, fish, eggs, tofu and pulses (such as peas, beans and lentils).
- **Dairy foods** such as milk, cheese and yoghurt, all of which contain calcium.
- **Healthy snacks** such as yoghurts, dried fruits, oatcakes and rice cakes.
- **Iron-rich food** Pregnant women can become deficient in iron, so make sure you have plenty of iron-rich foods (red meat, bread and green vegetables), and try to eat these with a glass of juice that has vitamin C, such as orange juice, as this helps the body to absorb the iron.
- **The odd indulgence**, but less is always more on this front.

What to avoid:

- **Cheeses such as Camembert, Brie, and soft blue cheeses** are made with mould and they can contain listeria, a type of bacteria that could harm your unborn baby.
- **Pâté** Avoid all types of pâté, including vegetable. This is because pâté can contain listeria.
- **Raw or partially cooked eggs** This is to avoid the risk of salmonella, which causes a type of food poisoning.
- **Raw or undercooked meat** Barbecued food is often a culprit here.

- **Liver products** This is to make sure you don't have too much vitamin A, as having too much means that levels could build up and may harm your unborn baby.
- **Raw shellfish** This is because it can sometimes contain harmful bacteria and viruses that could cause food poisoning.

What to cut down on:

- **Junk foods** such as biscuits, sweets, crisps and cakes. They are high in fat and sugar with little or nothing on the nutrient front.
- **Fast food** such as takeaways, burgers, pizza are all high in salt, sugar and fat.
- **Processed food** such as ready meals are high in salt and sugar even if it's fat-free.
- **Fizzy drinks** such as colas are high in sugar and the diet versions high in caffeine and additives.

What about fish?

Eating fish is good for your health and the development of your baby, so should be a part of your pregnancy diet; however, you do need to avoid certain types of fish, such as swordfish and marlin, and limit the amount of tuna you eat to no more than two tuna steaks a week. This is because they could contain high levels of mercury, which could affect your baby's developing nervous system. Also, have no more than two portions a week of oily fish, including mackerel, sardines, salmon, trout and fresh tuna. This is because these types of fish can contain low levels of pollutants.

Weight gain: what's healthy, what's not?

In a world obsessed with thinness, obesity and celebrity motherhood, it's easy to forget that gaining weight in pregnancy is a normal and essential part of a healthy pregnancy. Not only does pregnancy weight gain feed your baby's growth and development but it also enables you to have enough energy to deal with the changes taking place within your body.

"I've always worked hard to control my weight, but being pregnant threw that all out of the window. I was too sick to exercise and all my body craved was pasta and cheese. I used cry because I felt so terrible about my body. Finally, my mother said that my first responsibility wasn't to fit into my clothes but to make sure my baby was OK."

Anna, 31

Yet, despite this, many pregnant women find weight gain difficult to accept and become anxious, upset and downright depressed. And, as their weight increases, they begin to feel that they are either losing control or are in danger of becoming big for life. Part of the problem is that pregnancy weight gain usually goes on all over your body, not just your bump, something people never really warn you about.

Alongside this, water retention can puff you up, making you feel even bigger and more bloated. All bad news if you're aiming for a positive body image.

The good news is that gaining a huge amount of weight in pregnancy isn't an inevitable part of being pregnant. Gone are the days where the advice was to 'eat for two, and rest up', now the expert advice is for daily exercise and a healthy diet, both of which are the keys to the right kind of pregnancy weight gain.

How much weight you personally need to gain over your pregnancy depends on a variety of factors including:

- Your pre-pregnancy weight.
- Your body mass index (BMI) – an equation that works out if your weight is in the healthy range for your height (your midwife should work out your BMI at your first booking appointment at the hospital).

If your pre-pregnancy BMI was in the normal range (18.5 to 24.9), ideally you should gain between 11.3kg (1st 11lb/25lb) and 15.8kg (2½st/35lb) in your whole pregnancy, which is around 900g (2lb) to 2.25kg (5lb) in the first trimester and about 450g (1lb) per week for the rest of your pregnancy.

If you were underweight before becoming pregnant (a BMI below 18.5), you should aim to gain 12.7kg (2st/28lb) to 18kg (2st 12lb/40lb).

If you were overweight (a BMI of 25 to 29.9) you should gain 6.8kg (1st 1lb/15lb) to 11.3kg (1st 11lb/25lb).

If you have a BMI of 30 or higher, you should gain no more than 6.8kg (1st 1lb/15lb).

If you're having twins you should gain between about 15.8kg (2½st/35lb) to 20.4kg (3st 3lb/45lb).

tip

> If you were overweight before getting pregnant, or are worried that you are gaining too much too fast, speak to your midwife about your fears and let her help you.

Although this may sound like a large amount of weight to gain, understanding how this weight is distributed can help to alleviate your worries:

3.4kg (7½lb) is the approximate size of your baby at birth
680g (1½lb) is the weight of the placenta supporting the baby
1.8kg (4lb) is increased fluid volume
900g (2lb) is the weight of the uterus
900g (2lb) is breast tissue
3.2kg (7lb) is down to maternal stores of fat (vital to store nutrients and protein for feeding your baby)
900g (2lb) for amniotic fluid
Equalling a total of 13.6kg (1st 12lb/26lbs approx)

Gaining more than the recommended amount of weight, however, may do more than dent your self-esteem, as excess weight puts both you and your baby at risk of problems, such as gestational diabetes and high blood pressure, as well as labour complications. Gaining too little weight is also problematic, as it leads to an increased risk of delivering a baby with a low birth weight, who is then more likely to experience asthma, respiratory tract infections and ear infections as a child.

tip

Women who gain between 25–35 lbs during pregnancy, and who exercise regularly (but moderately) throughout pregnancy, are the most likely to lose their baby weight in the months following birth.

How much extra food do you really need?

Despite the myths, experts advise that you do not need to radically increase the amount you eat to support your growing baby until the third trimester, when only an extra 200–300 calories a day are needed. This is because the body works super-efficiently during pregnancy, and you'll find that you will gain only a few pounds in the first trimester and after that a steady weight gain of around 450–900g (1–2lb) a week for the last six months (depending on your starting weight).

How to relax about your pregnancy weight gain

- The weight gain only lasts nine months, which means you can lose it post-baby.
- You do not look fat. You look pregnant.
- Being stressed actually makes you crave unhealthy food, so relax and you'll eat more healthily.

How to have a blissful and relaxed pregnancy

In these time-starved times, most of us, even the most ardent of lazy girls, can find it hard to relax, chill and bliss out. Yes, we all know how to stay in bed, laze about and do nothing, but physically learning how to let go and relax is something else entirely. Yet, knowing how to bliss out is vital during pregnancy, partly because pregnancy is tiring and exhausting, but also if you don't let go every now and then you're going to feel shattered inside and out. It's also important because knowing how to relax is vital for labour.

fact

> Pregnant women who live highly stressed lives are far more likely to deliver prematurely than non-stressed pregnant women.

The good news is, there are ways to learn to chill, and these techniques can help you to feel more in control, less tearful, more energetic and happier all round. Here's how to do it:

Spoil yourself

By that I mean spoil yourself with pampering sessions that allow you to look after your body and bliss out at the same time. You may not be a girl who does this in normal life, but it can help restore your self-esteem and your energy levels in pregnancy. Try a day spa, or a manicure or pedicure, or even a special pregnancy massage.

Load up your iPod/MP3

You don't have to listen to whale songs and tinkling bells to relax to music. Choose whatever helps you to zone out and enjoy the moment, because this is what relaxing is all about: finding something that takes you away from worrying and stress, and allows you to relax.

Give swimming a go

This is your chance to feel weightless, no matter how big you are! Swimming is not only a massive stress reliever but an ideal exercise for pregnancy because, as well as being relaxing, it gives you a good workout while the water supports your weight.

Try Hypnobirthing or meditation

Hypnobirthing and meditation are forms of self-hypnosis, relaxation and breathing techniques that can help you relax during pregnancy, help you avoid pain relief during labour and help you to get through childbirth. These are techniques where you are aware of what's happening to you (you're not in a trance eating onions or pretending to be a rabbit), but you are able to tune out worries and distractions and just relax. To find out how to do it you either need to do a class (see Resources) or buy a CD and book.

If these techniques aren't for you (and not everyone fancies the more alternative route) a very simple way to relax at home is to turn off your mobile, Twitter, laptop and social networking sites for 30 minutes every day and lie down on the sofa. Being in constant touch with everyone may be your way of unwinding, but it won't help you to relax and let go. Go techno-free and just close your eyes and breathe; it will bring you closer to bliss than your beeping phone.

Also, do yourself a favour and learn to say no. For many pregnant women this can be the hardest thing to do, especially when it comes to friends and family, but it's the number-one way to give yourself some much needed time to actually bliss out.

Lastly, find a quiet place to zone out when you are feeling overwhelmed. A bath, reading a good book, a walk in the park, or even locking yourself in the toilet can help you to relax and zone out.

Remember, once the baby comes you will have less time to relax and bliss out, so the more you do now, the more energy you will have to cope with what's to come.

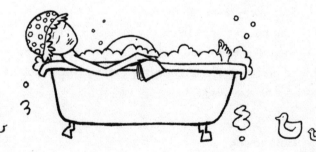

20 ways
to be healthy when pregnant

1 Maintain your posture

Extra weight gain changes your centre of gravity, and so to compensate for backache and sore calves you may find yourself contorting into all sorts of shapes in your efforts to stay comfortable. Keep your posture by wearing low heels and imagining a string pulling you upwards from the back of your head.

2 Revel in your amazing body

It takes a very healthy body to sustain a pregnancy, so even if you feel anxious about your changing looks, revel in the amazing thing your body is doing.

3 Step away from the mirror

Your bump, lumpy bits and whatever is irking you will only be magnified if you look in the mirror all the time. You're pregnant, you are naturally getting bigger, you have to learn to accept this.

4 Get moving

Researchers who studied 230 women during and after pregnancy found women who exercised during pregnancy felt less depressed about their bodies and happier with their pregnancy look.

5 Pamper yourself

Be sure to pamper your pregnant body: get a manicure, get your hair done, or go for that massage! These things can go a long way to making you feel better, relax and de-stress.

6 Avoid toxic people

That's people who are constantly complaining or miserable. Stress can be contagious, so avoid the transmitters who can make you feel blue and down.

7 Breathe more slowly

Breathe in through your nose and out through your mouth. Inhale deeply, count to five, then exhale slowly, counting to five. Do this five times once a day while sitting down, to help relax your muscles and nerves.

8 Be aware of where you hold tension in your body

Try lowering your shoulders, and stretching to help you relax, especially if you spend a lot of the day sitting down.

9 Pay attention to your feet

It sounds strange, but your feet can take a real hammering during pregnancy, as well as getting super-dry skin. Massage cream into them once a day – better still, ask your partner to do it for you!.

10 Don't focus on celebrities

Famous people's pregnant bodies are not the norm during pregnancy! Apart from the fact that many are born into the lean and slim body type, most have trainers, cooks and nutritionists working to keep them slim during pregnancy.

11 Drink more water

As well as needing to drink more fluids when pregnant, drinking water can stop you retaining fluid and feeling bloated.

12 Health and beauty is a state of mind

Meaning, if you're feeling blue and down about yourself, seek reassurance from your best friends, family and loved ones. So what if you're being needy – you're pregnant.

13 Pregnancy weight goes on all over

It's not what you're eating but just the way body fat lays itself down. The good news is that, seven months to a year after you've given birth, if you've been eating reasonably and exercising moderately, the fat goes away.

14 Don't over-exercise your tummy area

Apart from it hindering labour (your stomach muscles need to be able to relax in between contractions), pregnant bellies will not go flat post-birth. It takes time for your tummy to look smaller, so be prepared to have a pregnant-looking belly for at least a month after your baby is born.

15 Get some food advice

If you're stuck for what to eat, or don't feel like eating at all, speak to your midwife for tips on what to choose. Little and often is the best advice, with healthy and balanced meals over high-fat sugary ones.

16 Don't flunk the pregnancy food rules

You may feel it's being over-careful to avoid certain foods, but be aware that when you are pregnant, your immune system does not function as well as usual, so you are more susceptible to the germs responsible for food poisoning.

17 Give yourself a break

Although exercise is encouraged during pregnancy, if you can't face it or your body just can't cope with it, give yourself a break. Instead, aim for 30 minutes of activity a day – walk to the shops, do some at-home stretching or simply go to your local swimming pool and relax in the water (perfect in the last trimester when your bump feels horribly heavy). Everything you do counts (see below).

18 Make household chores count too

Get your heart pumping with your domestic-goddess duties. Outdoor work counts, too. Mowing the lawn is a great way to burn calories. Raking strengthens your arms and back, and digging works your arms and legs.

19 Back pain and pregnancy go hand in hand

Help yourself by paying attention to how you sit and stand. Sit with your feet slightly elevated. Choose a chair that supports your back or place a small pillow behind your lower back. Change position often, and avoid standing for long periods of time.

20 Watch out for iron-deficiency anaemia

Fatigue can be a symptom of iron-deficiency anaemia, but adjusting your diet can help. Choose foods rich in iron and protein, such as red meat, poultry, leafy green vegetables, wholegrain cereal and pasta, beans, nuts and seeds.

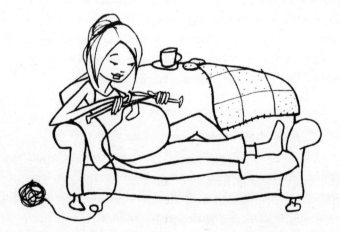

CHAPTER FOUR

Pregnancy looks

The truth that no one wants to admit aloud is that during pregnancy one of the areas that often deflates confidence levels is the radical and often swift body changes that come with being pregnant (probably because it feels too shallow and silly to say). Apart from noticing on a daily basis how much bigger you are getting, the running commentary about your size by friends, family and work colleagues can dent even the most solid of self-esteems.

fact

Seventy-eight per cent of women say they have concerns about how pregnancy and motherhood will change their weight and bodies, but 57 per cent won't discuss it with friends or doctors for fear of being thought shallow.

Alongside this maybe you've noticed other body changes that have rocked your confidence: perhaps your hair has got dryer, or your skin more greasy and blotchy, or perhaps, as I've said in Chapter 3, your body seems to be gaining weight everywhere. Whatever is happening it's probably making you feel somewhat ugly. What's worse is when you do tell others how you feel they probably say, 'Don't be ridiculous all pregnant women are beautiful', or 'Well, what do you expect, you're pregnant?' Neither of which helps much, because the truth is while some pregnant women look amazing, and some glide through pregnancy effortlessly not all pregnant women look and feel amazing, and just because you look worse for wear doesn't mean you have to put up with it or pretend it isn't happening just because you're pregnant.

If you're a high-maintenance kind of lazy girl, the chances are you have always scheduled in looking after your body and looks, so in pregnancy you're unlikely to be any different, unless of course your confidence has taken such a knock you've given up. If, however, you're so low maintenance that you don't get your legs waxed until the hair pokes through your 60 denier tights, then this chapter is for you, because the truth is if you want a blissful pregnancy you've got to learn that during pregnancy you have to take care of yourself.

Why? Well, for starters, feeling at odds with your new body and looks kills your self-esteem, which in turn ruins your confidence and makes you someone who is desperate for constant reassurance. It's not a pleasant place to be and not a happy nine months for anyone, least of all your best friends and partner. So here's what you need to know about getting to grips with your pregnancy looks.

Pregnancy fashion: how to look good with a bump

What's difficult about pregnancy is that your body is changing so quickly and you haven't had that kind of change since puberty. This means it's hard to have a stable body image and feel great about your looks and body, especially in the second and third trimesters. What's more, if you're not blessed with a trophy husband, you probably can't afford to be the doyenne of the maternity fashion world, splashing out every week on the latest new trend.

"Just when I think I've nailed looking good, I wake up and seem to have expanded in a different direction, or what felt comfortable yesterday is too tight today, or I'm too hot/too cold."

Kelly, 31 (six months pregnant)

Yet, maternity fashion has come a long way in just 20 years. Gone are the floral pregnancy smocks your poor old mum had to wear to hide her shape, and gone are the specialised old-fashioned shops. These days alongside your trendy maternity boutiques are high-street brands from M&S, to Gap and H&M selling affordable and fashionable maternity wear. The rules have also changed; where once it was deemed unfitting for a pregnant woman to show off her bump and cleavage, nowadays it's positively welcomed to show off your pregnant shape with tight-fitting tops and, dare I say it, sexy looking clothes.

It's all good news, even if you're at odds with your growing body, because it means there is something out there for everyone, and there is just no excuse to live in your husband's T-shirts, baggy joggers and pyjamas for nine months.

Of course, it's difficult trying to think what might look good when your body has changed so dramatically, so here are the lazy-girl pregnancy fashion rules.

Wear maternity, not plus size

This is perhaps the number-one rule when you're pregnant. Maternity wear will always suit you better than just going up a size, this is because maternity clothes are designed to fit your normal size with consideration for your bump and breasts. This means they will fit you properly on the shoulders, arms and hips and not leave you looking as if you're sporting someone else's clothes or lost beneath a sack of material. Plus, all maternity clothes have room for an expanding belly and allow for the additional weight gain, so should see you through at least two trimesters.

tip

Oversized jumpers and T-shirts will just make your shoulders look droopy and ensure you look heavy not pregnant.

Buy maternity clothes at the right time

In the first trimester, although your clothes will begin to feel tight and you may feel fat rather than pregnant, you can get by in slightly baggier clothes and elasticised waistbands. It's wise not to buy maternity wear now because (1) you're unlikely to know what pregnancy shape you will be; and (2) the clothes you buy now won't make it through three different seasons of pregnancy. However, from four months, maternity clothes are perfect, not only will they make you feel like a normal human being but they will also make you feel much more comfortable.

Buy maternity wear that is adjustable

Many dresses, tops and jeans are styled with adjustable parts to take up the extra material before you need it. This is perfect if you're on a budget and don't fancy shopping for clothes every four weeks. Remember, it may seem HUGE now, but you'll be filling it out by the third trimester. Also, try to buy wardrobe staples (see below) that take into account the seasons and the fact that you'll probably be wearing them post-partum to save money.

Always try things on

What suits you when you're pregnant is all down to the way you are carrying your baby. Some women look amazing in T-shirts and skinny jeans, as their bumps are small or they are tall, whereas others look more glamorous in dresses or skirts. The trick is not to try to second-guess what you're going to look like, and to always try on a range of clothes and styles so that you get used to what suits you as a pregnant woman and what feels comfortable.

Choose longer, darker tops

They not only accommodate a growing bump (which tends to pull tops upwards) but also streamline you to make you look longer. Think tunics and T-shirts to wear over jeans and leggings. Likewise, think colour, as dark shades help to make the upper body look leaner, while prints and bright shades draw the eye away from large bumps.

Accessorise

Now is the time to go for it on the accessory front. Think shoes, bags, jewellery, hair accessories and corsages. Good mum tips are:

- Wear designer sunglasses, says Lynne, 30, 'I can't wear anything fashionable, so these are my big comfort buy.'
- Buy a big leather shopper, says Natalie, 27, 'I've always wanted one, and now it's going to double up as a nappy bag.'
- Sian, 36, says, 'Big earrings, sexy jewellery and great shoes draw the attention away from always having to talk about my bump.'

Consider all the variations of pregnancy jeans and trousers

Like tops that cling to the breasts, or skim over or hold under, the best pregnancy jeans are also a matter of personal taste.

The maternity styles you can get all mirror the regular styles you can buy on the high street, with the only difference being the waistband. The options are: under-the-bump jeans (where your jeans and trousers settle just below your baby bump), over-the-bump jeans (an elasticised panel sits over the top of your bump), or jeans with expanding sides (they look normal from the front but have elastic at the sides to expand with you).

Which style you choose depends on what suits you best and what you feel comfortable with, although bear in mind that over-the-bump can be hot in the summer and under-the-bump a bit too breezy in winter.

Don't wear high heels

Celebrities make wearing high heels when pregnant look effortless; what you don't see is them soaking their war-torn feet later or being carried home by their PA. The fact is, as much as you may love them, high heels and pregnancy just don't go hand in hand. This is because, as your weight increases, and your body shape and centre of gravity change, your weight is thrown forwards, putting pressure on your lower back. Heels only exacerbate this motion, leaving you in a few hours with lower back pain and a painful throbbing in the ball of your foot (a bit like walking on sharp stones). Save high heels for special occasions when you can kick them off in the car on the way home.

How to dress for your changing shape

Are you having a pregnancy style crisis? If so, you're not alone. Fifty per cent of pregnant women say they have no idea how to dress well in pregnancy, with 20 per cent saying they just live in their husband's clothes. If you want to look good, the good news is you can. So here's a helping hand.

Problem You're all boobs, with a small bump.

Wear tops with open vertical necklines, which will give you more shape than T-shirts and help you to look more streamlined, rather than big all over. The aim is to try to make yourself look longer and less top-heavy, so also try empire-style tops and dresses. These are dresses that fit under the breasts and then skim downwards. Wrap dresses are also good, as they accentuate the cleavage but then skim downwards.

Avoid high necks and clingy tops.

tip

> Forty per cent of women take a D cup or above before they are even pregnant, so make sure you get fitted for a pregnancy bra.

Problem You're all bump.

Wear tops and dresses that float over your tummy and skim your hips. Try to steer clear of separates like a skirt and top, as these tend to make you look more pregnant if you have a big bump. Long tunics over jeans and dark trousers add length and streamline your look. And dresses also flatter. Empire lines are good, and straight-legged jeans, as opposed to leggings, will balance your lower body and will draw the eye away from your bump.

Avoid tight-fitting dresses and tops that you feel hold you in, and bias-cut dresses. These will only make your bump look bigger.

tip

Relax about your bump size. The baby aside, the size of your bump is also affected by the size of the placenta, how much weight you gain, the strength of your tummy muscles, and the amount of amniotic fluid you produce.

Problem You look fat, not pregnant.

This feeling often has a lot to do with a broad body shape (or the fact that you may have been overweight before pregnancy) and the fact that you are retaining water, which pumps up your arms and legs, making you feel bloated and fat. The good news is you do not look the way you imagine, but dressing well can help you to feel better.

Wear three-quarter length sleeves or loose bell sleeves to make your arms appear longer and more streamlined. Dark trousers and jeans also help you look longer. As for clothes, aim to create a shape, rather than hiding under shapeless tops and dresses. Think well-fitting shirts, deep V-necks and dresses that wrap around you to show you're pregnant and not weighty.

Avoid baggy tops, sleeveless tops and loose joggers. These just make you look heavy, not pregnant. Steer clear of tight T-shirts, especially ones that cling around your arms, and skinny jeans that look like a second skin on your thighs; if you're carrying excess fluid (which is often why you feel fat, not pregnant) they make you look weighty.

fact

Fifty-one per cent of women aged 20–39 are classified as overweight or obese before pregnancy.

Problem You're petite with a bump.

The chances are that if you're petite, any size bump will make you look very pregnant.

Wear styles to make yourself look longer. Keep styles simple and make sure all your dresses and skirts end above the knee. If anyone can afford to wear an ultra-clingy top or show a lot of leg it's you, as straighter shapes suit your tiny frame.

Avoid long styles that will drown you. Wide belts and baggy tops make you look like you're trying too hard. Also avoid big prints that look as if they are swamping you.

fact

Although it's true that the size of your baby is related to your own birth weight, your husband's genes also have an influence.

A lazy girl's guide to maternity must-haves

Belly band Also known as a bump band, this is a soft, wide fabric that comes in different colours and prints and sits over your bump, helping you to extend T-shirt lengths and hide unbuttoned trousers.

Bra extender A small extension panel that enables you to wear your normal bras for as long as you want (or until your cups spill over).

Maternity bra You won't need this until your cups start to squeeze you and you feel you can't breathe. Get fitted at around week 12, and again at the very end of the last trimester so that you can buy a nursing bra.

tip

> You will need to shop for a nursing bra again after you have had your baby because your bra cup size can jump two more sizes when your milk comes in.

Swimwear You may be in the 2 per cent of women who are able to get away with a thong bikini, but if not, invest in maternity swimwear, it's supportive and won't leave you embarrassed when you jump in the pool.

Flat shoes Your feet get a battering when you're pregnant due to the excess weight you're carrying, so opt for flat and low heels.

A large scarf worn around your neck can disguise an early pregnancy at work, and can be useful as a cover-up when breastfeeding in public as well as keeping you warm.

Nightwear You may sleep naked and feel very happy about it, but if you're suddenly rushed into hospital, it pays to have a nightdress (with front-fastening for breastfeeding) and a dressing gown handy.

One glam pregnancy outfit, because the chances are you'll be invited to at least one wedding/birthday/christening in nine months.

One smart pregnancy suit for work events.

One lazy pregnancy outfit Yoga workout gear is good here, as it doubles up as TV clothes and fitness clothes.

Pregnancy beauty: how to maintain your looks the lazy way

We all know what being pregnant does to your stomach, but most of us don't consider the way it effects all of our body parts, from our skin to hair to nipples and even vein damage and shoe size. Here's what you need to know.

Skin

As any teenager going through puberty can tell you, hormones, especially fluctuating levels of hormones, will affect your skin faster than you can say 'horrible spot'. During pregnancy your skin is going to see a lot of action. On the positive side, pregnancy can make your skin look dewy, young, fresh and plumped up – and will have all your friends begging for your secret. On the downside, you may be facing a myriad of skin problems that can leave you feeling at odds with your looks.

tip

When you are pregnant, your body produces 50 per cent more blood, resulting in more blood circulating through your body. This causes your face to become brighter and gives you that pregnancy glow.

Problem 1: stretch marks These are one of the most talked about skin changes that can occur during pregnancy. Almost 90 per cent of pregnant women will experience stretch marks, which appear as pinkish or reddish, or even purple, streaks running down your abdomen and/or breasts. Rubbing in lotions have been said to help in the prevention of stretch marks but this isn't proven, and in any case stretch marks occur because your skin is stretching to accommodate your bump, not because your skin isn't supple (skin is naturally supple and stretchy). Whatever you do, rest assured it will fade after your pregnancy is over.

One word of warning As your skin stretches and tightens, it naturally feels itchy and uncomfortable; however, if you begin to experience severe itching later in your pregnancy (possibly accompanied by nausea and vomiting) see your doctor; this could be a sign of something else entirely: a serious condition called cholestasis, which is related to the function of the liver and needs urgent medical attention.

Problem 2: acne Blame your hormones, especially in the first and second trimesters, when inflammations may well erupt. The good news is that as your pregnancy continues the acne will go away, but in the meantime topical medications like benzoyl peroxide or azelaic acid are safe to use during pregnancy. Oral medications, which are usually prescribed for acne, however, should be avoided during pregnancy, as they can harm your baby.

Problem 3: dry skin This is often down to dehydration. During pregnancy you need to drink at least eight 225ml (8fl oz) glasses of water a day (more than this is even better). This is essential because you need the water to supply your body with the liquid it needs to maintain your high pregnancy blood volume, and replenish the amniotic fluid that surrounds your baby.

tip

Drink a glass of water every half an hour. If you don't drink enough, all the fluid you drink will be diverted away from you to the baby, leaving you with dry and flaky skin and cracked lips (other signs include a dry mouth and feeling lethargic).

Problem 4: chloasma Also known as the 'mask of pregnancy', this causes dark splotchy (red, brown or pink) pigmentation spots to appear on your face. These spots most commonly appear on your forehead, nose and cheeks and are a result of increased hormones, which cause an increase in your skin pigmentation. Nearly 50 per cent of pregnant women show some signs of the chloasma, but the good news is it does go away. In the meantime, protect your skin with a sunscreen, as chloasma gets worse, and sometimes even appears for the first time, if you expose your pregnant skin to the sun without any protection.

Problem 5: sensitive skin Once again, blame your hormones for this. Fluctuating levels can cause outbreaks of eczema, impetigo and even hives. If you feel your usual creams are making things worse, try a dab of calamine lotion to calm things down. If any rash or irritation is painful, or it begins to weep and/or lasts longer than a week, see your GP for advice.

Hair

There are many things written about what you can and can't do during pregnancy when it comes to your hair. Although it's up to you to do what you feel is best, rest assured that there is no evidence to show that having your hair highlighted/dyed/straightened or even permed will harm your baby.

However, what's important to know is that nothing changes your hair like pregnancy. You may find your once fine hair becomes thick and luscious or drier than normal, or maybe even frizzy, and most of this is down to pregnancy hormones and the fact that your hair growth has changed. So, don't do anything drastic to your look, because post-delivery your hair will change again and it will take six months to revert to its normal condition.

What you also need to know is, thanks to the hormonal shifts of pregnancy, hair goes into a resting phase where it doesn't fall out (look in the plug hole when you wash your hair if you don't believe me); this means thicker-looking hair all through your pregnancy. The downside is that post-pregnancy and post-breastfeeding your hair will suddenly start to fall out in what seems like massive amounts (don't worry, you're not going bald, only entering a big falling-out period to make up for the pregnancy phase).

Hormones will also affect your hair's condition, so the best thing to do in the meantime is to have regular cuts and consultations with your hairdresser to ensure you're using the right treatments and treating it correctly.

Body hair

Although you may love the thick, luscious hair on your head, you may be horrified at all the new places your body is growing unwanted body hair.

"During my pregnancy, body hair started growing on my cheeks and skin. I became obsessed with tweezing them and even talked to my doctor about laser treatment. He reassured me it was normal – not that that helped my body image much."

Sam, 31

Again, it's those good old hormones that cause unwanted hair growth on the face – upper lip, chin, cheeks and even the neck – and also your back, breasts, nipples and abdomen. Although the pattern of hair growth should return to normal within six months, it's not much consolation if you feel you're turning into the hairiest woman alive. Hair removal is always an option, although don't do anything drastic like laser removal, as the hair will eventually return to its normal growth levels.

Troubleshooting: how to deal with those pregnancy body changes

Body changes galore happen throughout pregnancy. Many are the result of the physical impact pregnancy has on your body, and many are part of the development process of turning you into a feeding machine once your baby is born. The bad news is that some of these changes can seem alarming and freaky; the good news is that they disappear after delivery.

Body sweat changes

During pregnancy your metabolism increases, which is why you feel warm and sweat easily, especially when travelling or when the weather suddenly changes. The answer isn't more antiperspirant but wearing clothes that help to absorb the sweat.

Help yourself by choosing sweat-absorbing fabrics, such as cotton, that make you feel cool and comfortable.

Bump changes

Having a pregnant belly is not like having a fat belly, and the fastest way to learn this is to wear something too tight around your belly or to try to bend down to do your shoes up during the third trimester. The bigger your bump gets the harder it will become and the less give you'll have when you bend down. Apart from it being uncomfortable if you press this area (with too tight clothes or by bending), it will leave you feeling breathless and nauseous.

Help yourself by constantly paying attention to your pregnancy clothes. What fitted and felt good in the second trimester may not in the third.

Nipple changes

Bigger nipples – you're not imagining it; as your breasts grow, so do your nipples. In fact, as your pregnancy progresses, your nipples become larger and darker. You may also notice small, goose bump or pimple-like white areas on your areola.

These are normal and are known as Montgomery's tubercles and are harmless.

Leaky nipples – it sounds vile, but you may start producing colostrum any time after 16 weeks of the pregnancy. Colostrum is the first fluid a woman's breasts produce prior to milk and it is a clear or creamy-yellow substance that doesn't hurt or smell bad. It is the first 'milk' your baby will drink in the first few days after it's born. If you are leaking colostrum you may need to wear breast pads inside your bra. If the fluid is at all worrying or has a strong smell, see your doctor for advice.

Help yourself by wearing a bra that fits. If your nipples are sensitive, think about a slight padding in your bra, or nipple shields in your bra cups if your breasts are leaking colostrum.

Tummy changes

You may notice a dark line down your tummy from your belly button to your pubic bone in the second trimester. This is known as linea nigra and occurs due to the stretching of the abdominal muscles. It's all down to extra pigmentation in your skin and it will go away a few weeks after delivery.

Help yourself by not being too conscious of this, as no one will see it. If you're going swimming, choose a high-waisted bikini bottom or a swimsuit rather than your usual choice.

Veins

Varicose veins Usually the domain of the elderly, varicose veins are those bulky bluish veins that appear on the legs during pregnancy. Varicose veins can be uncomfortable and sometimes painful, and are more likely to appear if you have a family history of varicose veins. To help avoid them:

- Try not to stand for long periods of time.
- Walk around as much as possible to help the blood return to your heart.
- Always prop your feet up on a stool/Swiss ball or table when sitting.
- Sit with your legs higher than your head for at least 30 minutes a day.
- Avoid excessive weight gain.

Help yourself by Wearing support stockings. These are not the torture instruments you imagine but normal-looking tights in various deniers that have extra elastic support weaved in. They are available from all good department stores.

Spider veins are minute reddish tiny blood vessels that branch outwards and can be found on your neck, arms, legs and face. These spider veins are caused by the increase in blood circulation and do not hurt, and they usually disappear shortly after delivery. If not, laser treatment can help remove the veins that have not faded away. To help avoid them:

- Increase your vitamin C intake.
- Do not cross your legs when sitting, as this can exacerbate spider veins.

Help yourself by having a make-up consultation. Your skin changes a lot in pregnancy so your usual make-up may not be doing a good enough job. A consultation will take into account the coverage you need and the way your skin has changed.

Haemorrhoids are varicose veins in the rectum and frequently occur during pregnancy, partly because your blood volume has increased and also because your uterus puts pressure on your pelvis, making the veins in your rectum get bigger. Haemorrhoids can be extremely painful, and they may bleed, itch or sting, especially during or after a bowel movement. See your doctor and midwife for haemorrhoid cream.

Help yourself by eating a fibre-rich diet and drinking plenty of fluids daily.

Shoe size

You're not imagining this – your shoe size really does change during pregnancy due to the extra fluid in your pregnant body that tends to pool in your legs and feet by the end of the day. Many women experience swelling in their feet, and may even have to start wearing a larger shoe size. It's a pain, but don't rush out and buy a new shoe wardrobe, because the effect does go away post-labour.

Help yourself by wearing flip-flops if it's summer, or if it's winter wearing trainers or sport shoes. In the latter stages of pregnancy, you may prefer to wear slip-on shoes to avoid having to bend down to put them on.

20 *ways*
to feel body confident when pregnant

1 Invest in good underwear

This is your pregnant body's external support system. Buy a well-fitting pregnancy bra, pregnancy pants (above or below your bump) and a pair of support tights (amazing help with aching pregnancy legs and vital if you're on your feet all day).

2 Consider your beliefs about pregnancy

We all have a vision of what we'll look like when pregnant, what we'll do and how we'll never be like X who gained 3st and spent nine months on the sofa; however, until you're pregnant you don't know how your body is going to respond, so give yourself a break if you're too sick/tired/fed up to live up to your pregnancy ideal. Aim to be good enough, not perfect.

3 Join a mothers-to-be group

Whether it's a parenting class, pregnancy yoga or a breastfeeding workshop, hanging out with other pregnant women is liberating on the oh-my-god-what's-my-body-doing front!

4 Squash your competitive gene

It won't help during pregnancy and will either leave you feeling smug or crushed. All bodies are different, and no matter how you start out, your hormones will dictate how you feel and how you look.

5 Focus on the bigger picture

On low self-esteem days, concentrate on your baby's development and growth. Your body is changing in order to help your baby. It is a natural and amazing process.

6 Consider your pre-pregnancy body image

Research shows that women who have had a bad body image before pregnancy tend to have a worse one during pregnancy. Help yourself by paying attention to what's influencing your feelings; is it media depictions of pregnant women, the magazines you are reading, and/or the celebrities you admire? Only you can say.

7 Work on being positive about your body

Find one thing that you like about your body and accentuate it. It will give you a confidence boost. Whether that's a new cleavage, a firm but round stomach or even glossy flowing hair.

8 Have a sex life

It will make you feel good about your body and increase positive feelings about your new look. If sex is out of the question, make sure you increase how much you are touched by having hugs and even pregnancy massage. It will increase your endorphin levels and help you to feel better about yourself.

9 Police what you say to yourself

If you're consistently negative about your pregnant body, then that's how you'll end up viewing your pregnancy. Try to balance up what you say by adding one positive remark to every negative one.

10 Talk to someone sooner rather than later

Low self-esteem during pregnancy has a direct impact on how you will feel post-pregnancy when you are a mother, so take action. Talk to someone you trust about how you're feeling or seek professional advice and help from your midwife or doctor.

11 The tiredness and confidence link

Confidence always takes a major hit when you're tired and exhausted, so think about when you feel at your lowest about yourself and correlate it to your energy levels. Things always do look better in the morning.

12 Keep telling yourself 'This too shall pass'

It's an important mantra to remember both in pregnancy, labour and motherhood! Whatever horrible phase you're in, it's just a phase and it will pass.

13 Ask for reassurance

So you don't want to be needy, beg for compliments or be the girl who can't make herself feel better. On the other hand, we all need other people, especially those who love us and see the best in us. Let them in, they really will make you feel better.

14 Remind yourself you are more than your pregnancy

You're still a good wife/friend/daughter/employee who has her own talents and skills – don't erase who you are just because you're pregnant.

15 Educate yourself about pregnancy and motherhood

The more you know about what's going to happen to your body and when, the more in control you will feel and the more confident you will be.

16 Be daring with your pregnancy wardrobe

The good news about having a pregnant bump is that you can get away with a lot during pregnancy, such as body-clinging tops (remember for once your body is firm not flabby). Experiment with styles, colours and clothes you'd usually avoid.

17 **Resist the urge to wear your partner's clothes**
You deserve to look great during your pregnancy, and wearing clothes not cut to flatter your sexy new figure won't give you the confidence you need.

18 **Wear your bump with pride**
Don't try to disguise it, cover it up or drape things over it. You're only going to be pregnant for nine months and will probably show for only six of those so make the most of it!

19 **Don't compare bump sizes**
It's the cardinal sin of pregnancy and one designed to either have you feeling smug or depressed.

20 **Beware of the sun**
Many women find that during pregnancy their skin is more sensitive and that they are much more susceptible to sunburn and excessive skin pigmentation. So use more sunscreen, cover up in direct sun and avoid the sun where possible.

CHAPTER FIVE

Baby worries

Apart from the joy and euphoria being pregnant brings, having a baby also comes with its own special package of lazy girl anxiety and worry such as, 'Will I be a good mother?' 'What if I don't like it?' 'What on earth should I be buying?' and perhaps the biggest concern of all, 'How will we ever afford a baby?'

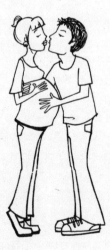

"The whole process of having a baby is anxiety ridden, simply because there are constant hard choices to be made, whether it's about screening tests, what kind of delivery to have, whether to stay in work or not, or what's the best kind of care for your child."

Natalie, 30, mum to Ellen, 3, and Cassie, 9 months

Although some of this anxiety is fuelled by the fact that having a child is an unknown quantity that as a first time parent you can't yet comprehend, much of the baby anxiety is made worse by countless adverts telling you what you 'have' to have when you're pregnant, as well as other parents spilling their financial and parenting horror stories. And let's not forget the tales in the media of how much it costs to bring up a child over a lifetime, how good/bad it is to be a working mother and how nursery ruins/makes your kids.

So the first thing you need to know (and remember) is that babies and toddlers are very simple creatures. They need food, warmth and love, and they don't care if they are dressed in the latest designer gear, whether their nursery/bedroom looks like a magazine spread and what pushchair/stroller/pram they are being taken around in. They also don't care what you wrap them in, the brand of their nappies and whether the toys you buy them are new or not. So, if having a baby has cost someone you know a fortune, or has someone you know tearing their hair out because Baby X will only wear cashmere and drink organic milk, you have to remember that these were choices the parents made.

Of course, at the same time you can't get away from the fact that having a baby does cost in terms of loss of income and childcare. There is no getting away from the fact that whether you decide to be a stay-at-home mum or a working mother, your salary is going to be decimated. But don't despair, it's not the end of the world: (1) You will cope because, let's face it, you have to; and (2) What other parents don't tell you is that you will save money, because having a baby (at least for the first six months) means relatively little social or shopping time.

As for the worry, well sadly that's just part of parenthood (ask your parents), and in time you not only get used to high levels of it but also learn to put your worries in perspective so that you can actually enjoy having a child. The good news is that being a parent is tough on everyone, so sharing your anxieties and fears is not only liberating but also a guaranteed way to help you realise that you're not alone.

Financial worries and your baby

fact

The average cost of raising a child to the age of 21 has crashed through the £200,000 barrier for the first time (to £201,809 to be precise) with parents typically shelling out £9,610 a year to feed, clothe and educate each new member of the family.

Before baby, how much you spent and what you were earning probably wasn't much of an issue. Perhaps you would have liked more (who wouldn't?) but it's unlikely you woke up in the small hours fretting about how you were going to cope with everyday life. The unfortunate by-product of being pregnant is that suddenly finances become centre stage in your life, as you start adding up the cost of having a baby, looking after a baby and taking time off from your job.

"We can't afford to give up work, but we also can't afford to pay nursery fees. I am pretending it's all not happening so I don't have to face it head on."

Tricia, 25

Perhaps, like many mothers, you'll wish you hadn't blown quite so much money on clothes/holidays and make-up? Or wish you'd saved more, or not been quite so quick to get credit cards and fill them up to the brim. Whatever your financial starting point, the important thing is to work forwards from here, not backwards. Yes, having a child adds up over a lifetime, but what people don't tell you is that on a day-to-day basis having a baby doesn't cost that much. Breast milk is free and the chances are you can beg and borrow most of the baby equipment. Even the stuff you have to buy won't break the bank if you shop smartly (see below).

On top of this, depending on where you live, there are benefits, tax breaks and one-off payments (see box on page 123) that can help you buy the necessities, take time off and pay for childcare.

Unfortunately, while now is not the time to change jobs (you may well lose out on maternity benefits if you change jobs while pregnant), now *is* the time to plan ahead, not only for how you'll cope when you are not earning a full salary but also what you will do at the end of your maternity leave.

Step 1: draw up a budget

Getting your finances in order early in your pregnancy really helps, because once the baby comes you'll be too busy to sort anything out. Plus it's crucial to have a financial plan that gets you through your pregnancy and then plans for the future when you're on maternity leave and when you go back to work (or choose not to).

The very first thing to do is make sure you're on the same page as your partner. This means discussing your ideas about childcare, spending habits, debts, bills and how you're going to cope with a smaller income for a few months to a year. Your budget should take into account your incoming money, including your maternity benefits, and your partner's wages, and all your outgoings – rent/mortgage, debts, bills, food and clothes. The aim is to ensure you have enough money to live on while you're at home with the baby, and enough money for all of the above and childcare costs (if any) when you're back at work.

Help yourself by:

- Knowing exactly how much your income will decrease by when you're on maternity leave and how you'll face this shortfall.
- How much childcare in your area will cost if you go back to work. Check out prices for private and state nurseries, local childminders, mother's helps and nannies.
- Cutting back on how you spend your income before the baby is born.

Step 2: don't panic if the numbers don't add up

It can be frightening to see in black and white how little money you will have post-baby; however, don't panic or think you're making the wrong decision to have a baby, because there are ways to cut back and make more money. Firstly, think about all the ways you can reduce your outgoings. Consider consolidating credit card and loan payments, swapping to a zero per cent credit card, changing utility and insurance companies for lower premiums and getting rid of unnecessary payments such as satellite TV, or two mobile phone bills, and so on.

"We saved about three hundred a month just by watching how much we spent on takeout food and at restaurants."

Lisa, 33

Secondly, make lifestyle changes by downsizing your habits; change supermarkets and buy non-brand over brand products, get your hair done more cheaply, don't buy clothes, make-up and toiletries all the time. Have a no-gadget-buying rule and basically reduce what you spend on a week-by-week basis, and you'll be amazed at how much you save.

Next, think about how you can make and save money before the baby comes. Could you take on a part-time job, work evenings or do some overtime? How about making money on the side with a home-based business? Try selling your old stuff online, or making something, or even offering babysitting services. Remember, every little counts.

Help yourself by:

- Asking for expert help, if your finances are in dire straits (see Resources).
- Shopping about online for everything, from insurance to utilities to supermarket products.
- Making savings, no matter how small, everywhere you can.

Step 3: claim what you're entitled to

Now is the time to check out what maternity benefits you are entitled to (see box on page 123), whether it's via your human resources department, your written job description or, if none of those help, what government benefits (if any) are available to you.

Depending on where you live, pregnant women are entitled to a whole range of free health care and sometimes even grants. Maternity leave is also protected in most countries; that is, you're entitled to come back to your job at the same level after taking time off with your baby, and you're entitled to take X number of months off to look after your newborn. If your company doesn't have a maternity package, then state benefits are available in most countries. What's important is to get informed and find out what you are entitled to well before you need to apply, as forms need to be filled in, notice needs to be given and certain medical certificates have to be collected from midwives and doctors. Help yourself by:

- Getting informed about what you're entitled to.
- Not feeling bad about claiming – you're entitled to child benefits and tax credits if you have paid tax.
- Applying for what you need at the right time and in the right way.

tip

There is a lot of bureaucracy and red tape around claiming maternity benefits, so if you want to be paid, pay attention to what signed certificates you need (to prove you're entitled and pregnant) and when you need to make your applications by.

Claim all you are entitled to

In the UK

Apart from a range of maternity benefits when you're
on maternity leave (check with your midwife and your
employer), there is child benefit, which is currently
given to children until they are 18 in the UK. However,
in 2013 this is due to change and will not apply to
children who's parents pay above the basic rate of tax
(currently over 44,000 pounds a year). Alongside this
if you're on a low income, or single income there are
various grants and allowances (for instance, you may be
entitled to free milk, fresh fruit and vegetables, infant
formula and vitamins vouchers under the Healthy Start
scheme) that can help you buy much needed essentials
for your baby. Legislation is changing all the time
so you may still be entitled to some grants and help
whatever your financial status in 2011 and 2012. Check
www.direct.gov.uk for up to date information.

In Sweden

Parents get 480 days off fully paid after the birth of
a child. Most of this is on 80 per cent of normal pay,
but many employers top that up to 90 per cent. Each
parent must take 60 days each, but how he or she
chooses to divide the remaining 360 days is up to
them, and the time off is valid until the child is eight
years old.

In Australia

The first perk is the baby bonus paid on the birth of a
child. You must make the claim within 26 weeks of birth

and meet Australian residential requirements. The tax-free money is paid for each child, so you would double for twins, and so on. The baby bonus payment is also available should your child be stillborn or die shortly after birth.

In Canada

Canadian maternity benefits include both a component for leave and compensation. Based on where you live, you may qualify for anywhere from 17 weeks to 52 weeks of maternity, parental or adoption leave from your place of employment without concern about losing your job. Additionally, the Canadian government may pay as much as 55 per cent of your normal pay, up to a weekly maximum, during a portion of your leave.

In Germany

In addition to the protected maternity leave, a period of parental leave may be taken until the child reaches the age of three. Since January 2007 new laws have come into effect whereby the former child raising allowance (*Erziehungsgeld*) has been replaced by an allowance for parents (*Elterngeld*). *Elterngeld* is assessed as 67 per cent of the net income of the mother or father (the average of the previous 12 months before the birth) up to a maximum monthly figure. *Elterngeld* is paid for a period of 12 months, or 14 months if both parents take leave to care for the baby. The aim is to encourage fathers to take time off to care for their children.

Step 4: don't fall into the overspending trap

Everyone wants the best for their baby, not only for their baby's sake but often to show the world what a caring and – let's face it – cool mother they are. Hence the sale of celebrity endorsed pushchairs, designer baby togs and products that are just a waste of money. If prior to being pregnant you adored shopping, branded products and buying, then the chances are you won't be much different when you're pregnant and a mum. However, now is the time to get your spending habits under control because, even if you're not a shopaholic, buying baby clothes, toys and baby paraphernalia are all ultra-tempting. Plus, because you're buying for your child, it's the perfect excuse to buy: you get your high without the guilt because you can justify that they'll 'love it/need it/look adorable in it'.

The only problem is that wanting to buy nice things for your child never goes away. In fact as they get older you will do it more and more, and this time under the guise that it's educational/everyone else has it/and they love it. All of which means you need to get a grip on your spending now before your child arrives and makes you bankrupt. Help yourself by:

- Thinking about why you're spending. Are you trying to buy a lifestyle? Make up for what you didn't have as a child? Satisfy your urge to shop, because you know you're supposed to be cutting back?
- Reminding yourself that you are buying for you, because your baby doesn't yet want anything.
- Not confusing what's necessary with what's cute.

5 ways to save money with babies

1. **Buy baby stuff on eBay** Babies grow notoriously fast and most mums do everything they can to stop their houses turning into a warehouse of used clothes, hence selling baby stuff lock, stock and barrel at bargain prices on eBay.

2. **Beg and borrow** Anyone who has ever been a parent will have baby equipment they are willing to lend or give you. Give it the old once over first to make sure it's in good condition and never borrow bottles, mattresses and dummies/soothers.

3. **Try Freecycle** for larger baby toys (baby gyms), furniture (cots, Moses baskets and bouncer chairs). You'll be amazed at the good stuff people give away.

4. **Don't give up work until you have to** Maternity benefits are often time-limited (depending on who you work for and where you live), so the longer you can stay in work, the more money you'll have when you're off.

5. **Breastfeed** It's cheaper than formula and you don't need endless bottles and teats.

The baby products to-buy list

Having said this is the time to save money and cut back, you can't get away from the fact that you do have to buy some baby-related products; however, you can stop worrying about what to buy, because what you actually need is less than other parents would have you believe. In fact, for the first two months, all a lazy girl needs is:

- Lots of maternity pads and breast pads (for you)
- Nappies
- Babygros – go for newborn and bigger, as who knows what size your baby will be when she is born
- A baby blanket and a warm suit and hat (newborns get really cold)
- Car seat
- Pushchair/pram
- Moses basket/cot
- Bottles and teats (for expressed breast milk and/or formula feeding)
- A steriliser
- Muslin cloths – a necessity for drooling babies

Once you have sleeping, eating, clothing, changing and transporting covered, everything else you buy is extra. Having said that, buying is not always so cut and dried. So here's what else you need to know about buying baby gear:

Car seats Buy new, not second-hand, as a car seat that's been in one accident may not protect your baby in another, and you can't always tell by looking if it's damaged. Plus, damaged car seats aren't uncommon; a survey commissioned by Sainsbury's discovered one in ten second-hand car seats currently in use in the UK had been involved in an accident. Also, get your car seat fitted properly, firstly to see if the model you're buying actually fits in your car and, secondly, to ensure you know how to put it in safely.

Crib and cot mattress Government health bodies and health officials advise the use of a new mattress with every child. A mattress you have used for a previous child, or been given by someone else, however well looked after, carries the risk of introducing your new baby to bacteria and mould. Also, an older mattress will not provide the same comfort and support that a newer one will give.

Pushchairs View pushchairs carefully and make sure you check the folding mechanism and raincover, and whether the seat reclines (essential for sleeping babies). Also, ensure that you know how to put it up and down and that it will fit on public transport. One very well-known brand of pushchair does not fit down a bus aisle, which means it has to be folded before getting on – a huge pain in the rain and when it's busy. Also, check that a folded pushchair will fit in the boot of your car (many won't if you have a compact car) and that it's not too heavy to lift.

tip

When buying a pushchair, test out whether you can open and close it with one hand, how heavy it is and if it fits into your car.

Baby bouncers and walkers Check for safety. Do they topple easily? Do the clasps all work? Is the material clean? Are the straps in good working condition?

Nappy-changing table or tray (to be placed over a cot) You may think you'll just do the changing on the bed or sofa, but believe me your back will soon rebel. It pays to buy a baby-changing mat and either a tray or table so you can change your baby without giving yourself chronic back pain.

Second-hand buys

"eBay is fantastic for baby clothes, toys and equipment. People often sell products in packages for around a tenth of the original price."

Caroline, 32

Baby clothes You can buy these cheaply online, through baby sales or you may even be given them by friends. Beware though that once you have a baby you will stockpile an amazing amount of clothes, and many people can't wait to dump everything, lock, stock and barrel, on some poor mother-to-be. Be selective, ask for specific items and don't be afraid to say no to clothes.

Baby toys Apart from the basics, you pretty much won't know what your child wants to play with until he arrives. So to stop your home from turning into Toys R Us, say no to all toys until your baby arrives.

"Initially I gratefully accepted two baby walkers, as I'd read that kids loved them, but Kim wasn't interested at all. She preferred to walk on her own holding on to furniture, so the walkers sat in the corner cluttering up our flat and collecting dust."

Janine, 32

The non-essentials

There are many, many things you will be led to believe you need for a new baby, and much of it is about a lifestyle choice rather than what a baby needs. For starters, you do not need to have a beautiful nursery full of toys, books and educational DVDs. Babies play with relatively little, and to begin with aren't interested in much besides sleeping and eating and you. By the time they want toys and books you'll find you've been given plenty or can borrow them from the library.

Likewise, they don't need much besides a bouncy chair or play mat (and a rug will do just as well as a mat). It's also way too early for a highchair. A baby sling is optional and feeding bowls, baby towels and swaddling blankets are all unnecessary, as you can use what you already have in the house.

"I really liked the idea of a baby sling, and this cool baby pram for the baby. We spent a fortune on two wonderful products only to find the baby hated the sling and wouldn't go in it and, because he was so long when he was born, he outgrew the pram in months. I can't believe the money we wasted."

Carly, 28

Baby products are also a waste of money. Read through any catalogue and you'll find ranges of products designed to make your life as a mum easier (and your purse lighter) but in all reality, although many work fantastically well, they aren't necessary. Plus, until your baby is here you won't really be able to work out what he or she wants and needs, because every baby is different.

Childcare decisions and fears

Apart from worrying about your pregnancy and all the accompanying health fears that come with having a baby, the other area of worry that's likely to be plaguing your mind is what to do about work and childcare.

The reality is that around seven out of eight mothers now work and, according to a report published in the UK, the number of stay-at-home mothers has dropped by a quarter in the past 15 years. In 1993 there were 2.7 million full-time mothers in the UK; the new research estimates that the figure will fall below 2 million by 2010. The survey concluded that most parents work because they cannot afford not to. That, in a nutshell, is the dilemma you're probably facing while being pregnant and, while you probably won't have to decide what you're going to do for sure right now, it pays to consider it earlier rather than later.

tip

When it comes to working mother versus stay-at-home mother, the earlier you start thinking about it, the more of an informed choice you'll be able to make when the time comes.

Whether you'll be a stay-at-home mum or not is dependent on a lot of factors, not just whether you can afford to. Lazy girl questions to discuss with your partner are:

1. **Can we afford it?** This means can you, as a couple, afford to live on one salary alone or one full salary and a part-time salary? Will the money cover all your basics and any possible glitches along the way, and what will you do if a sudden redundancy/illness or job loss occurs? **If you only ask yourself one question, this is the one to ask and to know the answer to.**

2. **Do I want to be a stay-at-home mum?** Not all women are made to be stay-at-home mums. It doesn't make you a bad mother who doesn't want to be with her child, if you can't take the relentless repetition of caring for a very young baby. In fact, being a working mother if you miss it (or need the money) will make you a better, less stressed mother when you are at home caring for your child. Sometimes this is something you will only realise during maternity leave.

3. **Will my career survive a career break?** A very important question, because if you're going to lose income when you eventually go back to work, or find your career phased out, or even find it impossible to re-enter, you need to think about what other options are available to you, such as training, while you are a stay-at-home mum; perhaps a home business or even your current business on a freelance basis?

4. **What do we want to do about childcare if I work?** Do you want one-to-one childcare in your own home with a nanny? Or are you looking for a nursery place or a child-minder? If you know very little about any of these options, you need to research each and every one of them to make sure you understand the pros and cons of each (see opposite) and

then make your decision. Also bear in mind that although you should think about this now, once you have had your baby you will be able to know better what may work best for your child's personality.

5. **Can we find decent affordable childcare?** You may want a full-time nursery space or nanny, but can you afford it? Research this thoroughly, because childcare when a child is under two years is frighteningly expensive (about the same as private education is when they are older).

Childcare - your options

Who looks after your child when you're back at work is a scary prospect, and one that takes a certain leap of faith, gut instinct and the ability to not let mummy guilt get in the way of your judgement. What's important to know is that whatever you choose to do there is a report/research/fact out there somewhere that is guaranteed to make you feel like a bad and inept mother who is somehow damaging her child for life.

"I never read much about motherhood and babies before I was pregnant. Now everything I read scares me. I was going to go back to work after six months, but the papers say nursery care is a bad thing. Then again I read that not having a working mother is bad for your baby. What should I believe?"

Amy, 30

In just one week, the media recently reported three different studies: the first one saying how nursery before the age of two made boys aggressive and unhappy; the second one stating that children who were looked after by their grandparents were educationally behind their peers when they got to school; and the third, advocating that stay-at-home-mums were bad for their daughter's self-esteem. And all this is in just one week of reporting! So what is best for your child when it comes to childcare? The answer is: whatever you feel works best for you as a family, as there is no one perfect solution and no one perfect answer.

Nursery places

Pros Trained staff, long opening hours, you know where your child is at all times, plenty of feedback and children the same age for your baby to eventually be friends with.

Cons Hugely expensive and your child is often looked after by a fairly young nursery nurse at the mercy of older children. You don't always know what's going on and there is usually a waiting list to get in.

Help yourself by looking at how nurseries are regulated and approved. Visit all prospective places and ask for guarantees of training levels and a breakdown of costs. A decent nursery should be able to tell you all of this and more.

fact

More than 700,000 children attend nursery for more than four hours a day.

Nanny

Pros Trained one-to-one care. Tend to have references and will look after your child in your home (sometimes live in, sometimes not). You will have complete say on your child's routine and many nannies are flexible about hours.

Cons You don't know what they do when you're not there and they can be hugely expensive.

Help yourself by asking around for recommendations. A good nanny will be in demand. Know what you expect of her and be clear about how you want your child brought up in your house.

Mother's help/au pair

Pros Cheaper than nannies and nurseries; live in your home and help you around the house with cleaning and shopping, and with childcare.

Cons Not trained and tend to be very young, or are students who speak another language.

Help yourself by always taking references and having a trial period where you can watch what's happening.

Child-minders

Pros A registered childminder is a professional carer (but not a trained nanny, which is why they are cheaper) who works from their own home – and can provide your child with care in a family setting. Childminders have to be registered with the appropriate government regulatory bodies. When registered, they are checked for references, training, police record and health, and their home is inspected to make sure it's a safe and suitable environment for children.

Cons They look after one or more children of different ages, are not trained like nannies and work from their own homes. You have little say over your child's routine.

Help yourself by asking around and seeing what people can tell you about local childminders. Always view a childminder's home and ask yourself if the place is safe, clean and well equipped. Is it a place where your child will feel happy?

A grandparent

Pros The cost is minimal (if anything); you get a say about your child's routine and peace of mind that your child is with someone you trust.

Cons A very young child can sometimes be too much for an older person to cope with and your child may not get out and about enough with an ageing grandparent.

Help yourself by always having a trial period before you go back to work to see if your parent(s)/in-laws can cope and like the job.

Common baby worries

First-time pregnancy and parenting is a bit like going into an unknown land where everyone speaks a different language but expects you not only to understand what's going on but also to cope with it with a big smile on your face. Which is why if you're currently worrying about giving birth and motherhood, and all that it encompasses, you're not alone. Firstly, it's probably important to realise that everyone has common baby worries that are, well, important to consider before your baby arrives. Worries such as how will I cope, what will I do without sleep, what if I can't breastfeed, what if baby's head is huge? And so on. Working through these considerations in our head prior to giving birth can help us to cope post-birth; however, what's vital is to remember that you're just working through potential possibilities, not creating a blueprint for motherhood.

Should we find out the sex or not?

"I really want a boy"

Ally, 24

While some people are of the belief that it's good not to find out what you're having for the surprise value or because it makes you push harder at the end, there are valid reasons for knowing. Firstly if you or your partner have your heart set on a particular sex then knowing either way can help you come to terms with the sex of your child well before the birth (having a boy when you had your heart set on a girl or vice versa can cause bonding problems post birth). Certain genetic diseases also run in males or females so again knowing the gender can help here. Lastly, if you're an organised girl you may simply want to know the sex so you can buy the right clothes pre-birth.

You can find out the gender of your baby at your 20-week anomaly scan. However, be aware that sometimes the sonographer can get it wrong or won't be able to see the sex depending on how accurate the machine is and/or the way your baby is lying. Diagnostic tests such as Chorionic

Villus Sampling (CVS) and Amniocentesis will give you an accurate result, but these are serious tests and carry with them a risk of miscarriage and so should not be used just to determine whether you are having a boy or a girl.

We can't agree on what to name the baby?

"My husband wants to use an old family name, and I want something unusual and new, how do we agree on a name?"

Sam, 26

There is a psychology to names with some studies saying what you call your child can help or hinder his/her chances in school and in life. Whether this is true or not is hard to say, however, what is known is that trying to be too original, using a deliberate misspelling, or inventing and/ or abbreviating names in a 'unique' way are sorely regretted mistakes by parents and later by their kids.

Of course where you live will directly affect what you choose. In France the law prohibits all names except those on an approved list, while in Germany invented and androgynous names are banned as well as the influence of celebrities' children's names. It also pays to think carefully about how your baby's name will be abbreviated by his/ her friends, and think about the historical and well-known connotations of a particular name. Lastly consider how hard the name is to spell. Your little darling won't thank you if he's 25 years old and still having to explain/spell his/her name to others.

If you and your partner are totally stuck for a name you can agree on buy a baby book and systematically go through the listings, bearing in mind that when you see your baby you'll know for sure and if you don't you'll just have to pick one anyway or else be fined.

As for people not liking your name choice or trying to influence your name choice in an annoying way, don't disclose the name you love and want until the baby is born. This way annoying person number one can't say, 'I hate that name it reminds me of xxxx' and annoying person number two can't say, 'Oh I used to know a horrible person called X'. After all this is your baby and your name choice so don't let anyone make you feel bad about it.

What if I think my baby is ugly?

"I worry what my baby will look like."

Jules, 26

Worrying that your baby won't live up to the beautiful image in your head is more common than you think. Yes, it sounds shallow and foolish, but for many women it's a real worry. What you have to realize is a couple of things, firstly all newborns look well squashed and not so cute, and don't really come into their looks for a couple of weeks. Secondly, you will think your child is wonderful and gorgeous even if he's not because he's your child and represents you and your partner.

Look back at newborn pictures of yourself for verification and remember once your baby's personality comes into it, you'll be enrolling him into baby modelling because then you'll really see how gorgeous he is.

I'm terrified of giving birth

"What if I can't take the pain of labour?"

Pat, 32

Everyone worries about this, and it's not surprising because it's very rare to know you're actually going to be in a lot of pain for a long period of time and have to cope with it. Mostly, this is a fear of the unknown and is fuelled by other people's birth horror stories (a weird by-product of pregnancy is having people tell you scary birth stories). What you need to know is this: yes, labour is painful, but the pain comes in waves, meaning you get a break between contractions to catch your breath and recover. Without this recovery period no one would ever be able to cope with labour. Secondly, there are a variety of methods to help you cope with the pain – gas and air, lying in water, epidural, painkillers – all of which can either ease or take away the pain. Thirdly, the pain (which is really the powerful muscles of your uterus contracting and releasing to ease your baby out) is an essential and normal part of labour that you're built to cope with. You may not like the experience, but understanding it helps immensely.

Will sex be the same after giving birth?

"I worry that vaginal delivery is going to ruin my bits."

Frances, 35

One could easily come to the conclusion that after all the stretching of childbirth things will never be the same again down below. Which is why it's important to understand that the vagina is built like an accordion – meaning it's designed to stretch open and bounce back again, thanks to all the muscles. So, sex won't change very much in the feeling department, if you wait the approved time (usually six weeks, but your doctor will tell you what is recommended); however, it may well change in the libido and energy department thanks to baby tiredness.

What if I hate motherhood?

"My advice is to not have any preconceived ideas about what it will be like. I always felt I was made to be a mum, and fantasised about what it would be like and how I'd love to play all day and do painting with the kids etc. Then I had three babies and it was nothing like that. Talk about a shock to the system!"

Tricia, 35

Motherhood is a massive life change, and if you weren't worried about it even just a tiny bit, you'd be in danger of looking at it through rose-tinted glasses, which would be frightening. The reality is that not everyone loves motherhood. That doesn't mean they don't love their children but more that they find the everyday grind of being a mother hard and relentless. And in many ways, in the beginning, being a mum is a thankless task, as a young baby doesn't tend to respond very much. Later, it's hard because overwhelming tiredness takes over. The good news is it's not a crime to say you sometimes hate motherhood or worry that you will, because that's the message that comes across from many women.

Help yourself by lowering your expectations of the good and bad things that motherhood will bring. Talk to trusted friends (the positive kind) who can tell you the pros and cons, and even ask your mother. The trick is to be positive and realistic, and realise that you're considering all of this without knowing what it's really going to be like to have a child you adore, with it's own personality and charms.

Should I make the baby fit into my life or change my life for my baby?

"We swore a baby wasn't going to change our life, and for the first six weeks we took our son everywhere with us, even to the pub at nights. Then my mum pointed out that maybe he wasn't sleeping well and eating properly, and maybe I was so knackered because we were without any routine whatsoever."

Tina, 32

People without children love to boast that they won't let a small baby change their life. It's laughable, because nothing changes your life like a baby. A baby is helpless and needs lots of care, meaning you can't treat it like a friend that's come to stay or a pet that can be ignored in the corner. That's not to say you have to let it take over your personality and stop you having fun, but more that you'll save yourself a lot of grief if you adapt to it, rather than expecting the baby to adapt to you.

What if I turn into Mumzilla - the baby bore?

"I knew I'd become a Mumzilla when even my mum's eyes started glazing over when I talked about the baby."

Tracy, 30

Having a baby is a bit like losing masses of weight, finding religion or falling in love: for a while it's all you can think about, talk about and make your life about; however, hopefully, in time, thanks to friends and your returning sanity, you'll find your equilibrium again and make your life balance out. Mumzillas who don't, tend to be women with a competitive streak who have swapped their work competitiveness for competitive parenting or who have simply lost the plot when it comes to all things baby related.

Help yourself to avoid the Mumzilla trap by ensuring your life is about more than your child and your role as mum. Even if you just do one thing for yourself each week – go to the gym, take up a hobby, read a book – it will help you to keep your life in perspective.

What if my baby is HUGE?

"I've been told my baby is very big and it's scaring me. What do I do?"

Carly, 25

Firstly, doctors are often wrong about how big a baby is going to be, because of the way babies are measured. It's very rare for a woman to have a baby that is too big to pass through her pelvis; however, it can happen, due to problems such as

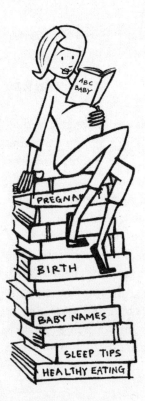

gestational diabetes and if your partner is very big (after all his genes affect the size of your baby as well as yours). If your baby is big, your doctor will spot it well before delivery and won't let you opt for a normal vaginal delivery, which may be problematic for you and the baby, but will probably suggest a C-section. Remember, the size of your bump isn't always the greatest indicator of the size of your baby, so listen to the medical advice you are being given. Here is a ray of light if your baby is big: a recent study found that large babies are likely to do better at school, have more stellar careers than small babies. So it's worth it in the end.

20 things
to know about babies

1 Babies don't cost as much as you think
Yes, over a lifetime your child will cost you a fortune, but in the here and now they don't cost that much, apart from nappies and milk (and if you breastfeed they'll cost you even less).

2 Your baby will sleep a lot in the first six weeks
And when I say a lot, I mean a lot. A newborn will sleep 16 hours a day or more, although not all in one sitting.

3 A baby won't smile at you until six weeks
Although they will mimic you smiling in the early weeks, their first proper social smile is around the six-week mark.

4 Newborns use a lot of nappies
For a small baby, they wee and poo a lot; expect between eight to ten nappies a day.

5 Babies don't see far, but they see a lot
Newborns only see objects within 20–25cm (8–10in) of them, but they delight in studying faces and patterns, particularly those with sharp outlines and stark light/dark contrasts.

6 Your baby's senses aren't fully developed at birth

Your baby's hearing will be fully mature by the end of the first month outside the womb, but the sense of sight develops gradually over six to eight months, at which point your baby will see the world almost as well as you do.

7 Your baby will recognise your voice from birth

In fact, your baby will recognise your voice even *before* birth. Researchers have long known that newborns recognise – and prefer – their mum's voice over anyone else's.

8 Don't panic about baby's racing heart

The heart of a newborn baby beats between 130 and 160 times a minute (about twice that of a normal adult). Plus, babies breathe much faster than adults – 30–50 times a minute compared to an adult's 15–20 times a minute.

9 Newborn babies are very strong

A newborn baby's grasp is so strong that if they grasp your finger, they can support all their body weight on that grip. This, however, fades with time.

10 Newborns have what's known as a walking reflex

It's also known as a stepping reflex. If you hold your baby upright, one foot 'steps' in front of the other as if he or she is going to walk.

11 Your newborn will demand to be fed a lot

Your newborn should be nursing eight to 12 times per day for about the first month and should never go for more than four hours without a feed, even at night.

12 Always put your baby to sleep on his back

Your baby should sleep on his back, as this is said to lower the risk of sudden infant death syndrome (SIDS), but when awake it's important to allow babies to lie on their front or sit up safely. If babies play on their front, their muscles will develop properly, avoiding the risk of misshapen heads. Always turn your baby on to his back if you find him sleeping on his front.

13 Dummies aren't as bad as you think

Settling your baby to sleep with a dummy can reduce the risk of cot death (SIDS), as it encourages her to keep breathing. Don't worry if the dummy falls out while your baby's asleep, and don't force a baby to take a dummy if she doesn't want it. Experts believe that if used for a short period of time it can aid speech development.

14 Babies like massage

A study found that when massaged daily, premature infants developed more rapidly than those who were not massaged. Normal-size babies also love to be gently massaged, especially along their back and legs.

15 Talk to your baby from birth

The key language-learning years for children are between birth and six years, and babies learn language through listening and speaking. Hearing you in conversations will be enough for baby to develop her own language skills.

16 Be careful of your baby's feet

A baby's feet comprises mostly cartilage (as the bone structure is still developing) with gaps between the bones. These bones are very soft and pliable – so pliable that even tight-fitting socks can misshape the toes. Shoes are only needed when your child starts walking.

17 Babies are born with swimming abilities

Babies can be born underwater, as they can naturally hold their breath; however, it's important to know that they lose this instinct shortly after birth, so don't throw your baby into water and expect him to know what to do.

18 Your baby already knows if she is left or right handed

It's decided as early as ten weeks gestation which hand your baby will favour over the other in life.

19 All babies have a button nose

You may be arguing who 'gave' baby the nose but all newborn babies have a pug nose, as the bridge of the nose isn't there at birth – it grows later.

20 Newborns don't cry tears

Newborn babies cry a lot, but they don't produce any tears. There is moisture to lubricate and clean the eyes but proper tears don't appear until the baby is between three and 12 weeks of age.

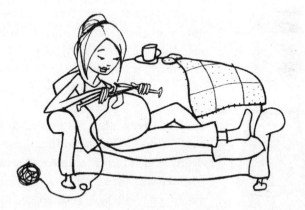

CHAPTER SIX

Birth day

Are you erring towards the 'too posh to push' scenario when it comes to giving birth, or wholeheartedly embracing the natural no-pain-relief method? Or are you like lots of lazy girls, pushing the whole idea to the back of your mind

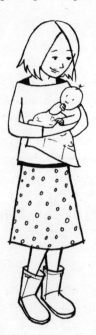

and refusing to think about what's to come and how you're going to cope? If you're going down the latter route, I can't blame you, because labour is not something that you should be spending weeks thinking (or, should I say, worrying) about. What you need to know is this: going into labour is rarely (if ever) a sudden thing that has you doubled over in pain with water gushing over the floor. Usually, contractions start slowly and build to a crescendo, hours (sometimes even days) later. Which means you will have time to get to the hospital (or wherever you're meant to be) and will have time to prepare yourself mentally for what's to come.

"I was constantly worried I'd be out and suddenly go into labour. When it did happen, I felt the contractions when I was driving, but they weren't so bad that I had to stop. They took about four hours to get to the painful kind and another three until we were ready to go to hospital."

Julie, 35

fact

The average time for first time labour is between 16 and 20 hours.

Having said that, it does pay to get informed about what happens during labour. Not only will this ease your anxiety and help you to feel more in control on the day but it also means you are more likely to have a birth that you feel happy with. Being informed means understanding the birth process, getting to grips with the medical terminology and knowing what your options are.

So, even if you're too busy to do anything else, make sure you:

1. Know where you are giving birth and why.
2. Understand the different ways you can give birth and write a birth plan.

3. Know what your pain-management choices are.
4. Find out how your body will aid the birth process.
5. Take a childbirth/parenting class and pick a birth partner.

Get all of the above right (and from the right sources as opposed to the over-medical or anecdotal ones) and you'll be able to make decisions all the way along that you'll be happy with, from what to do if you're overdue to the best form of pain management during labour.

tip

Don't watch footage of women giving birth. It won't help you with your own labour and it will just scare the pants off you.

1. Where to give birth and why

Choosing where to have your baby is a personal choice, even if sometimes it doesn't feel that way. What's important is to first know all the facts about the pros and cons of each choice and secondly to listen to what your doctor is advising you to do. This is because not all births are straightforward, and if you have a pre-existing condition or your pregnancy is at risk your safest and best bet is to have your baby in hospital. Finally, where you live and whether it's your first or second pregnancy will also impact on where you deliver your baby. Having said that, in general your main choices of where to have your baby are: at home, in a hospital delivery room, in a birth unit attached to the hospital or at a freestanding birth centre (not attached to a hospital).

A *hospital birth*

The majority of women choose to give birth in hospital, but even within a hospital setting you will still get a variety of choices and being there doesn't automatically mean your birth will be medical and assisted. For a start, many hospitals now offer the option of delivery in a consultant-led unit or in a hospital birthing unit.

fact

Ninety-five per cent of births take place in a hospital environment.

A consultant unit is part of a general hospital, and is staffed by obstetricians (doctors who specialise in birth where there are complications) and midwives. Here you are able to have all kinds of pain relief, medical help and assistance, but the room may be small and you may be placed on a monitor to check your baby's heart rate (and so restricted to the bed area).

A hospital birthing unit is also part of a general hospital but is a unit led by midwives only and has a much more at-home feel to it. It's primarily for women who want to give birth with little or no medical intervention with the emphasis in this type of unit being on birth without interference. You cannot have an epidural in this unit but you know help is nearby if you need it.

"I was really happy with my hospital birth. Halfway through labour I started to panic and my husband didn't know what to do. The midwife and doctor just took control of the situation and calmed me down, told me what to do and reassured me. I couldn't have done it without them."

Helen, 28

If you want a hospital birth, be sure to check out the hospital, the delivery unit and the postnatal ward (most hospitals do a new-parent tour) before you go into labour. This can help in a variety of ways. Firstly, it enables you to know exactly where to go when you're in labour and what the protocol is at the hospital. Secondly, it lets you get a clear idea of what the birth and post-birth environment will be like.

Why choose a hospital?

Well, it can make you feel safer and more relaxed if it's your first pregnancy, and it's ideal if your pregnancy has complications or you're worried something may go wrong and/or you're being induced. With midwives and consultants on hand all the time, you will be well looked after, although you may get a selection of midwives throughout your labour rather than just one.

The downsides are you may have to wait for a delivery room and an epidural, but at least you're in the right place.

Your hospital bag

This needs to contain what you definitely need to take to the hospital:

1. Your hospital/maternity notes
2. Your birth plan
3. Money for phone cards (in case you can't use your mobile)
4. A selection of baby clothes, blanket, car seat (though it's unlikely you'll leave the same day if it's your first birth or you have any complications so you may want to leave the car seat for your partner to bring in later), baby hat
5. Formula and bottles, if you're not going to breastfeed (as most hospitals won't supply these)
6. Lots of nappies
7. Healthy snacks and bottled water for labour
8. Flip-flops for the shower (believe me you'll need these)
9. Birth props such as a birth ball, your own pillow, and so on
10. TENS machine (if you're using one)
11. Toothbrush and toothpaste
12. Maxi sanitary pads for post-birth
13. Shampoo and soap
14. Nursing bra
15. Towels, nursing nightwear, a robe and slippers
16. Comfy clothes in case you're stuck in hospital
17. Magazines/books in case you're stuck in hospital
18. iPod/MP3

What not to take:

1. Valuables – you don't need to be worrying about these when you nip off to the shower
2. Your credit cards and purse (just take money with you)
3. Camera (get your husband to bring one and take it home with him)

Checklist: do I really want a hospital birth?

- Are you ready to be restricted about how much you can move about during labour?
- Can you deal with not having the same midwife with you throughout the whole labour?
- Will you be able to cope alone without your partner on the postnatal ward?
- Can you handle doctors/midwives who try to push your labour in a certain direction?

A home birth

As you might expect, a home birth literally means having your baby in your home. Studies show that having a baby at home helps to relieve stress and generally makes the birth more comfortable for you.

fact

Of all births in England and Wales in 2006, 2.7 per cent took place at home.

Studies also show that home births result in a more active birth (where you can move around and find a position that's comfortable) and are usually less likely to end in an assisted delivery (where your baby is helped out with a ventouse or forceps). Having said that, around 20 per cent of women having home births have to be transferred from home to hospital because of concerns about pain relief, a long labour or the baby being in distress.

"I want a home birth, but I'm worried because I am not the hippy type to use alternative medicine and candles and I worry that when the time comes I'll freak out."

Jane, 32

It's also important to bear in mind a number of things regarding a home birth. Although you may be more comfortable at home, you cannot have an epidural with a home birth, and drugs that are available at home will vary according to where you live, but usually include Entonox ('gas and air'), and pethidine, also called Demerol.

Next, you have to look for a midwife with plenty of home births under her belt; this means with plenty experience of handling potentially difficult situations. In certain countries your health authority will let you choose who you want but, if not, consider finding an independent midwife (these are fully qualified midwives who have chosen to work in a self-employed capacity). Make sure that whoever you choose has experience, and that you get on; however, be aware that in the UK independent midwives do not have indemnity insurance should anything go wrong (insurance companies will not sell it to them as there are too few independent midwives), which is something else to consider.

How to get ready for a home birth

1. **Think about where you will give birth in your house** A spacious room, rather than a bedroom is best to give birth

in, and being near a bathroom is also good. At the same time, think about which room you'll feel most comfortable in, especially if you have neighbours nearby, and consider what you'll do post-birth.

2. **Talk to your midwife or doctor about what you need** but it will probably include the following:

1. A waterproof sheet, old sheets and a stack of old towels are a necessity if you're giving birth on the floor or thinking of using a birthing pool.
2. Clean towels and blankets for post-birth.
3. A bucket for the placenta.
4. Pillows, birthing ball, bottles of water (to drink), snacks for all of you.
5. Sanitary pads for post-birth.

3. **Think about pain relief** There are plenty of pain-relief options for a home birth such as gas and air, pethidine, TENS machines, aromatherapy, and even Hypnobirthing. Think ahead about what you might want, and check that your midwife is experienced in any of the pain relief methods that you want.

4. **Think about your birth partners** Part of the pros of giving birth at home is that you can have a variety of people to support you; however, think very carefully about who you're going to choose and why. In most cases it's best to have two people and the midwife, but check with your midwife to see what she says.

5. **Practise with your birthing pool** If you're hiring a pool for a home water birth, then fill it as a test run before you go into

labour, because it might not be as easy to do as you thought or it may be too big for your room. You may also have to clean it.

6. **Have your hospital bag ready** Just in case you have to go to hospital, always have a bag ready with your notes at hand.

> ### *Checklist: do I really want a home birth?*
>
> * Will I feel safe and comfortable at home without a doctor present?
> * Can I cope without an epidural?
> * Can I deal with the post-birth mess?
> * Is my partner supportive of the idea and willing to help?
> * Is there enough space at my house to have a home birth?
> * Will we be able to cope alone together after the birth?

Birthing units

These independent units are situated away from hospitals where you are able to give birth in a home-away-from-home environment. Run by midwives there are no doctors present, and although lots of pain relief is available you will not be able to have an epidural and the emphasis is on little or no medical intervention.

Water births

Giving birth in water is now a recognised and encouraged part of labour because, essentially, being in water during labour can help you cope with your contractions, alleviate stress and even help with the second stage of labour (the pushing part). Most hospitals now have birthing pools as do birthing units, and you can hire birthing pools to use at home if that's where you're planning to have the birth; however, not all midwives or hospitals will allow you to actually deliver your baby in the water. This is because there may not be a midwife available who has been trained in caring for births under water, so always check first so that you won't end up disappointed.

2. Write a birth plan

Knowing all the different ways you can possibly give birth (see below) is important before you go into labour, because once you're in labour it's too late to find out the nitty-gritty details. Knowing your options is also important because it enables you to write what's known as a birth plan.

A birth plan is basically a list of how you would ideally like your delivery to progress, and it not only helps you to envisage what's going to happen but it also tells the midwife and doctor what your priorities are.

However, the key word is 'ideally' because childbirth doesn't always go to plan, so there's no point in saying, 'Absolutely no pain relief and no C-section', because if your labour turns into an emergency, this may be the only course of action. What your birth plan should really contain is details of:

1. Your birth companion and whether you want them to be there all the time.

2. Whether you have special cultural or religious needs that need to known.
3. What positions you'd like to try for labour, such as active or mobile, or whether you would like to be in the bed.
4. Whether you want to use the birthing pool.
5. Options for pain relief.
6. Skin-to-skin contact post-birth (see Stages of Labour on page 173 for more on this).
7. Vitamin K injection for baby (see Chapter 8).
8. Whether you intend to breastfeed.
9. What you'd like to happen in an emergency.
10. Whether you want students observing or not.

You can download sample birth plans from the Internet or just write down what you want on a piece of paper.

3. How you might give birth

There are three main ways to give birth:

Vaginal delivery

This is the most common way to give birth and refers to the normal delivery of your baby through the vagina with or without pain relief.

Assisted delivery

In about one in eight births, a baby needs assistance or help to be born. An assisted birth is where the midwife or doctor uses instruments (either forceps or ventouse) that attach to your baby's head so that she can be pulled out.

Forceps look like large tongs and have curved ends to cradle your baby's head, and the ventouse has a plastic or metal cup attached to a small vacuum pump, and a handle for pulling. The cup fits on top and towards the back of your baby's head.

Your midwife and doctor may recommend an assisted birth if:

- Your baby has become distressed and her heart rate has risen.
- You are too tired and can't push any more.
- Your baby has stopped making progress through your pelvis.

Caesarean section

This is an operation in which a baby is delivered by cutting open your abdomen and womb and removing the baby and the placenta.

fact

About 20 per cent of babies are born through Caesarean section (some emergency and some opted for).

Don't assume a C-section is the easy option. It may help you to bypass the pain of a vaginal delivery but recovery is longer and harder. You will have stitches so will find it hard to move around, and won't be able to drive or lift heavy objects for at least six weeks afterwards.

5 Reasons for an assisted delivery or C-section

1. **Placenta praevia** A rare condition where the placenta covers the entrance to the uterus.
2. **Foetal distress** When the baby's heartbeat speeds up, and doctors and midwives can tell she's in trouble.
3. **Breech birth** The baby is legs down, rather than head down and is unable to turn.
4. **Multiple babies** Twins can be delivered vaginally but if there are more than two babies they are delivered by C-section.
5. **Maternal problems** Perhaps a previous delivery was difficult or you're in some kind of difficulty.

4. What to do if you need pain relief

There's one fact of labour you can't avoid: it's going to hurt. So it's a good idea to start by thinking about what sort of pain relief you might like to make use of should you need it, and also when to ask for it. Here are the options you might want to consider:

TENS machine TENS stands for transcutaneous electrical nerve stimulation, and the theory is that the electrical pulses it makes prevent pain signals reaching your brain. It's said to work best in the early stages of labour, but some women say it does nothing for them. If you want to use a TENS machine you will need to hire one (see Resources).

Gas and air, otherwise known as Entonox, is composed of 50 per cent oxygen and 50 per cent nitrous oxide. You breathe it in through a mouthpiece or mask as soon as you feel a contraction starting. When the gas starts to make you feel a little light-headed, your muscles relax and you are no longer affected by your contraction. Some women swear by gas and air, others say it makes them feel sick and they don't like the light-headed feeling.

Being in a warm bath/birthing pool One great way to reduce labour pain especially if you're at home is to get into a warm bath. Not only will the water help lift the weight of the baby off of your back but it also helps to lessen your contraction pain and make you feel more relaxed. The same effect occurs later in labour if you use a birthing pool.

Breathing techniques Learning to breathe through your pain is one of the most effective ways to manage your contractions in the early stages of labour (and all the way through if you're opting for a natural delivery). Unfortunately, when we're in pain, the first thing we do is hold our breath until it passes, when it's actually better to take a deep breath as the contraction begins and then to slowly blow air out of your mouth through the painful part.

Epidural is a local anaesthetic, which is injected into a section of your spine to numb the nerves so you don't feel the pain of contractions during labour. It can be given early on in labour but not too close to the pushing stage/ second stage of labour, as it's more effective if you can feel the contractions during this stage. These days you are likely to get what's known as a mobile epidural, which allows you to move around and still use your bladder. The pros are it works within 20 minutes and you will receive effective pain relief without sedation. The cons are it can make labour longer and, in rare cases, a leak of spinal fluid may occur, causing a bad headache which will mean you need to lie flat for a couple of days.

fact

If you want an epidural, ask sooner rather than later because the chances are you will have to wait for it. There is usually only one anaesthetist on a labour ward at a time.

Pethidine is like morphine and works within 20 minutes of being administered; it is then topped up as needed. These drugs affect the whole body and although they don't interfere with labour, they can cause side effects including drowsiness and nausea. The downside is that the baby is also going to get these medications – some babies show signs of sleepiness immediately after birth.

Alternative therapies: homeopathy, acupuncture Although there is no proven scientific evidence to prove these alternative therapies work, there is plenty of anecdotal evidence. If you want to give them a try, speak to a practitioner and your midwife to see what is appropriate for you (see Resources).

5. How your anatomy will help you give birth

The body is an amazing machine made to help you grow and give birth to a baby, meaning whichever of the above options you choose, your body is going to aid you in the birthing process. The first thing you have to realise is that, despite the infamous 'squeezing a melon out of a pinhole' comment, this isn't (thankfully) what actually happens during labour.

Early labour starts with gentle contractions, which are the muscles of the uterus slowly and gently squeezing your baby downwards to make the descent towards the cervix. With this, your cervix starts to open and widen. It'll go from being closed to about 3cm (1¼in) or 4cm (1½in) dilated and may feel like the mild cramps you get with your period, or a dull ache or backache.

As the baby's head moves near to the top of your cervix, the cervix will start to soften and gradually flatten out to open to about 10cm (4in). This is wide enough to let the baby out and you are now what's known as fully dilated.

When this occurs (and this stage can take hours) your baby is ready to move down the birth canal. This has widened for him and become engorged with blood, pushing your bladder forward and your rectum backwards, leaving it open for your baby to travel through. What's more, the front of your pelvis is a joint, and this also opens up to give your baby more room to pass through.

All the way through your pregnancy, the hormone relaxin has been secreted into your body to loosen and soften your joints and ligaments, and this too can help your pelvis to expand during labour.

Furthermore, your baby's head has two soft spots, called fontanels, where the bony plates in his skull have not yet fused. This allows the bones to overlap and 'mould' to your body as it comes through the birth canal. As baby comes through the cervix and down through the birth canal he will turn so that the smallest part of the head comes out first (known as crowning), then his body will rotate (again to make it easier to exit the birth canal) so that his shoulders and the rest of his body can be born.

fact

Your birth position counts: where women have given birth lying down, the majority have said post-birth that they would prefer a different position next time. Women who have given birth in an upright position say they would choose an upright position for their next birth.

6. *Childbirth classes*

Many couples balk at the idea of taking a childbirth class, thinking it will be full of couples desperate to have a natural birth and women forcing you to use washable nappies and breastfeed. The reality is that although some can be like this the great majority are full of normal people who just want to find out the truth about childbirth and parenting.

"I'm glad I took the classes, it put my mind at rest about labour and about the choices I'd be given in hospital. The woman running the course also gave me some great tips on how to handle over-zealous doctors, which came in really handy."

Jo, 29

Depending on where you live there are a variety of choices when it comes to classes; some are free and paid for by your medical services and some are private. The latter are best if you're pushed for time and want to cram the knowledge into two days or less, and it's always better to do a local class. The reason why is you'll meet other pregnant women in your area who will be invaluable once you're at home with your baby. It's the perfect place to help put your fears at rest and also to find out who you can talk to if you're struggling with a problem (see Resources for details).

tip

Childbirth classes tend to focus on what happens during labour, pain relief, what to do if things turn into an emergency, and what happens post-birth, breastfeeding and early parenting problems.

7. Choose a birthing partner

A birth partner is an essential part of your labour process and the right person will be able to help you through labour, as well as calming you down, supporting you (both physically and emotionally) and making medical decisions for you if you're unable too. If you are having a hospital birth, you may be able to have two birth partners present, perhaps your husband/boyfriend and a friend or your mother. If you're at home you can have more, although bear in mind that less is more with birthing partners.

A potential birthing partner could be:

- The father of your child; however, if he doesn't want to be there (not every man can bear the idea of it) or you don't feel he will be able to give you the right kind of support, then you should choose someone more appropriate
- Your best friend
- A sister
- Your mother
- A doula (a professionally trained and independent caregiver who gives emotional and physical support during labour)

Experts argue over whether fathers-to-be should be present, but what's important is not what *they* think but how *you* feel. If you want your partner there, then tell him and be sure to also tell him what to expect (or let him read it for himself) and how you'd like him to help you during labour.

Some women just like their partners to be present, others want some hands-on help. Of course, you probably won't know until you are in labour, but give him an idea of what you may want him to do.

fact

Studies show that having a loving birth partner to support and look after you can make labour less frightening.

8. Other people's birth stories

Do you really need to hear other people's birth stories? Well, if they are positive and reassuring, yes, but if they are scary and frightening, no! The problem is that some people love to talk about their horrible birth stories and elaborate in such detail that they leave you white with fear. The reality is that for every horrible birth story there is a good one. Not everyone is treated badly, or rushed into surgery or left to cope without help. On the whole what you don't hear is that:

- You will cope with labour because millions of women do so every day.
- Labour is usually straightforward.
- You will have plenty of help along the way.
- In the weeks following labour you will forget all about it.
- Your baby makes the pain worth it.
- One day you will have forgotten all of it and will attempt to do it again!

So, in a nutshell, if someone starts to tell you a bad birthing story just shout 'NO!' and refuse to listen. Who cares if they are offended, if it's not going to help you, why do you need to hear it?

Are you really in labour?

By now you should know what labour is all about, what to expect, what happens and where you'd like to have your baby. All that's left now is to know the signs of being in labour. Everyone is likely to warn you about being in false labour or tell you that it's wishful thinking when you think labour is coming on. So, what you need to know is this: you know your body better than anyone else, and even if you haven't given birth before, if you feel as if you are in labour, or are worried about contractions you have been having before your estimated delivery date, speak to your midwife or doctor for reassurance. Other than that, here are the signs of being in labour:

Having a show

During pregnancy your cervix is closed with what's known as a mucus plug (a fair description of what it actually is), to keep out infection. Days or hours before labour starts your cervix will start to open a little, and the mucus plug will come out. This is called a show. It looks a bit like a mass of jelly and can be stained with blood. If you have a show and nothing else happens it's always worth calling your midwife/ doctor, because once it's out you are at risk of infection.

Regular contractions

Labour contractions are felt in the groin and in the lower back. They may radiate down your legs and thighs, be felt across your bottom and all around your pelvic region. These contractions are not sharp but dull and crampy, very like bad period cramps. In fact, many women feel contractions for weeks before they go into labour. They are mostly felt like a tightening across the belly and are known as practice contractions or Braxton Hicks.

To know if you are in labour you have to work out how strong and regular the contractions are. A full-on labour contraction is so strong that you will not be able to do much other than grab on to something and breathe while it's happening.

Contractions that are close together

To measure the contraction intervals, time them from the beginning of one contraction to the beginning of the next. Look for a regular pattern of three to five minutes apart. The usual advice is to call the midwife/hospital and make your move when they start to get this close.

Your waters break

If your waters broke with a pop or a gush, the contractions that follow will almost certainly develop into progressive labour. With a slow leak, contractions may or may not lead anywhere. Although be aware that you can still be in labour if your waters haven't broken (make sure your midwife and doctor know your water has broken or started to leak).

Feeling the need to go to the hospital

If you feel as if you really need to go to the hospital, then go. They will give you a check-up to see how you're progressing and if you're not fully dilated they'll give you the option to stay on a ward or go home and come back later.

What happens once you're in labour

While everyone's labour is different, what's important to know is the three stages of labour.

tip

When a woman tells you she was in labour for 72 hours, she's counting from the earliest stages of labour – not what's known as active labour (when you're 3cm dilated and your contractions are coming every five minutes). Don't let tales like this one worry you.

First stage

The first stage of labour is when contractions start to open up the neck of your uterus (cervix) and this stage consists of what's known as: early labour, established labour and the transitional phase of labour.

Early labour is when your contractions start gently but aren't close together and they aren't so painful that you can't walk, talk or generally carry on what you're doing at home.

Established or active labour is what the midwives time your labour from and this happens once your contractions start to come regularly, about once every three or four minutes, with each one lasting about 45 seconds to one minute. At this stage your cervix is about 3cm (1¼in) dilated and you'll need to get to hospital or call the midwife. Once labour is established your contractions will be painful and your cervix will open at an average rate of about 1cm (½in) an hour, depending on your body, the drugs you've taken for pain, and whether you are being induced or not.

The transitional stage of labour happens as you move towards the last centimetres of dilation, just before you begin pushing. It's called the transitional stage of labour because you will notice a distinct shift in how you feel. This is mainly as a result of high hormone levels that leave you feeling an emotional wreck as well as shaky and even nauseous. It doesn't last long (about 15–60 minutes) but you may well feel like you can't go on at this point, especially as the contractions start coming thick and strong.

Second stage

This is the pushing stage of labour, where you literally help to push your baby through the birth canal. Again, you will hear various time scales for this, with some babies popping out within 10 minutes and others taking an hour or more. What's important in this stage is to listen to your body and your midwife and not just push and push.

To begin with, you'll feel the pressure of your baby and then get a strong urge to push. With every push, your baby will move through your pelvis and then she'll slip back a bit. This is completely normal, and whether you realise it or not your baby is moving down the canal.

When your baby starts to reach the opening of your vagina you'll feel her head. At this point it's essential to listen to your midwife and go slowly so that your baby doesn't tear your vagina as she comes out. In some cases you may need what's known as an episiotomy (a surgical incision through the perineum made to enlarge the vagina and assist childbirth). This is done if the midwife feels the baby may tear you or if the baby needs to be born quickly or the birth needs to be an assisted one (medical experts also believe a small cut heals better than a forced tear).

At the end of the second stage your baby will be born!

Third stage

Before you have a baby it's easy to think the final stage of labour is when your baby is born, but it is actually when you deliver the placenta. This can be a natural or managed stage. Natural means your body expels it naturally. This can take up to an hour and you may have to push again. A managed third stage involves an injection that causes the uterus to contract strongly and the placenta to come away, so that it is delivered quickly. You do not have to push or do anything with a managed third stage, and it has the added advantage that you are at a lower risk of losing a lot of blood.

After the placenta and membranes are delivered, the midwife will examine your vagina and perineum to see whether you will need any stitches. If you do, these will be done right away.

What happens post-birth

Once your baby has been born, she will be placed on your tummy, while the midwife (or your husband) cuts the umbilical cord. Your baby will then be given what's known as the Apgar score. This is a test to evaluate a newborn's physical condition and to determine any immediate need for extra medical or emergency care. The Apgar score is usually given to your baby twice: once at one minute after birth, and again at five minutes after birth.

The Apgar score

Five factors are used to evaluate the baby's condition and each factor is scored on a scale of 0 to 2, with 2 being the best score:
1. Activity and muscle tone
2. Pulse (heart rate)
3. Grimace response (medically known as 'reflex irritability')
4. Appearance (skin coloration)
5. Respiration (breathing rate and effort)

Doctors and midwives add the five factors together. Scores are between 10 and 0, with 10 being the highest possible score. A baby who scores a 7 or above after birth is considered in good health; however, a lower score doesn't mean that your baby is unhealthy or abnormal but that she simply needs some special immediate care.

If the Apgar score is fine, then your baby will be laid on your chest for skin-to-skin contact.

tip

Skin-to-skin contact is usually given if the baby is healthy but sometimes your baby may need to be checked over first depending on what happened during labour. If you want skin-to-skin contact right away make sure it's on your birth plan and don't be afraid to ask the midwife for it.

You will then be left with your baby for a few hours to recover in the delivery room but observed at regular intervals until you are ready to go to a post-natal ward. You have to stay in this room, as post-birth complications do arise in women, with bleeding and bladder problems being common. The good part is you will finally be allowed to eat and drink something, get cleaned up and, of course, cuddle and even feed your newborn baby (if you're both up for it. For more on breastfeeding see chapter 7).

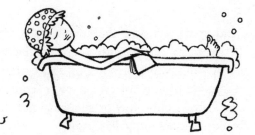

20 ways
to get through your labour

1 Don't panic
Easily said than done, but remember your body is built for this; millions of women do it every day and help is at hand for when things get too painful.

2 Trust your caregivers
... but at the same time don't be afraid to speak up, give your opinion or disagree if you're not happy with the ways things are going. Remember, it's your body and you have a right to an opinion.

3 Make sure you drink
Keep bottles of water with you all the time. Keeping hydrated is essential for your energy levels, which you're definitely going to need as labour progresses.

4 Keep moving
Gravity is your best friend during labour, so don't just lie down. Keep moving around the room, outside if you're able to (take your birth partner with you), and stay upright for as long as possible.

5 Play around with positions

Some positions aid labour, make contractions easier to bear and help speed things up. For instance, squatting helps open the pelvis area, while kneeling and standing (with help) allow gravity to do its bit. Play around with what feels comfortable for as long as you can.

6 Use the birthing props

Swiss balls (huge blow-up balls), birthing stools and cushions can all help you to feel more comfortable during labour. Give them a try to see what works best for you.

7 Bring your iPod

Music can help distract you during the first stage of labour. Don't be afraid to bring your iPod and block out the sounds of the hospital, as some studies say that music not only helps mums-to-be to relax but also to get in sync with their breathing.

8 Don't be body conscious

If you're a shy kind of person, the thought of giving birth can feel embarrassing. What you have to remember is that doctors and midwives have seen it all before and won't be shocked by anything. Don't focus on what's exposed; focus on getting through the labour.

9 Stay at home for as long as possible

Obviously, not until the baby's crowning, but at least until you are 3cm (1¼in) dilated (this is when your contractions speed up). Studies show that mums do far better being in their own environment with their own things than on a crowded and noisy antenatal ward waiting for things to happen.

10 Don't be afraid to ask questions

Not even the ones you're afraid will sound stupid. If you're confused, distressed, worried or just unsure of what you've been told, ask and keep asking. If you're too exhausted, make sure your birth partner is your advocate.

11 Watch what you eat

During labour, your stomach and intestines slow down, so you don't want to burden your sluggish digestive tract with heavy, fatty meals. Eat light foods that will give you energy.

12 Don't blame your partner for the pain

Yes, he got you pregnant but you wanted it too, and it's all too easy to take out your pain on your birthing partner. Be fair to him and let him sneak off for breaks now and again. It's really not easy to see someone you love in pain and know that you can't do anything for them.

13 Don't despair if you feel you can't go on

There comes a point in labour when you may feel that you truly cannot go on and just want someone to yank the baby out or knock you out. Usually this happens around transition when the first stage of labour is about to be over. This is the result of hormones (as well as exhaustion). Just hang on in there – you're nearly done.

14 When you're told to push, push as hard as you can

Not only will it help your labour along but it's also the only way to deal with the pain. Grunt, yell, scream – make animalistic noises, whatever it takes but PUSH!

15 Turn your mobile phone off

If you're in hospital you will have to do this anyway, but if you're at home the last thing you'll want is to be bombarded with texts and calls finding out how you're coping.

16 Keep wet wipes and ice chips nearby

Labour can make you feel horribly sweaty and dirty, and wipes can help you cool down and feel refreshed. Ice chips are perfect to suck on to stop your throat and mouth feeling dry.

17 Don't worry about what's happening at home

If you've gone into labour suddenly the chances are you're worried all is not ready for the baby at home. If this is the case, ask your partner to call someone you trust, such as your mum/best friend and ask them to go in and get the cot/Moses basket ready, tidy up and shop for some food for you.

18 Forget about bottom burps and bodily emissions

All that straining sometimes makes it happen during labour and midwives won't be shocked, they'll just clear it away super-fast. Just make sure your birth partner knows it might happen.

19 Try positive visualisation

If you feel a panic coming on, it really does help to visualise a peaceful scene (beach/grass meadow and your bed at home) and just breathe your way slowly through it.

20 Tell yourself that by this time next week it will all be forgotten

And it really will be, because you'll be too busy with baby to even think about what you went through.

CHAPTER SEVEN

Life after birth

The odd thing about being pregnant is that it's so easy to become so busily focused on the pregnancy and birth that you don't think very much about what it will be like when you bring your newborn home. Of course, like most mums-to-be you will have thought of the necessities, but beyond that, the idea of life with a small baby probably doesn't figure too much in your mind. That's things like: what to say to him, what to do when he is awake and basically how to get on with everyday life when you have a baby in tow and are probably on your own for the first time in ages.

The fact is that the first 12 weeks post-birth are a sharp learning curve of trying to work out what your baby needs, how all the baby equipment works, and how and when to do things with a baby.

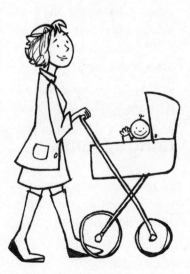

"I didn't realise how terrified I would be to do things like getting on the bus with the baby and pushchair, walking up the road or even just going for a drive with the baby, and this from someone who was used to travelling the world on her own. The first time I got on the train with the baby all by myself, I cried with relief when I got home."

Annie, 30

The fact is, it does feel scary when you first have to look after a newborn baby on your own and even if it's only for eight hours a day it can feel like 20 or more.

Although, in time, you'll get to know, love and adore each other, in the beginning being with your child can feel like a strange blind date. That's not to say you'll regret it but more that you'll find life with a baby hard to navigate. The good news is that once you get the hang of it it's easier than you think.

Coming home

At last after nine months and what seemed like an endless stay in hospital, you, your partner and your baby are home alone, the question is – what now?

"It was weird coming home. Suddenly my husband and I looked at each other and started laughing. We had no idea what to do or where to start with this little stranger in our living room."

Karis, 28

Arriving home alone, or being alone with your child once your family has gone home can be an unnerving experience. What can help is to walk round your house with your baby in your arms and to just chat to him about where you are. Of course, he won't understand you, but remember, if it's awkward for you, it's like being on an alien planet to him. Then just focus on keeping him warm, holding him and chatting, and everything will start to feel normal. Of course, the scary element of being trusted to look after this small baby is another thing entirely, but as a long as you take it one step at a time you will be fine. Potential difficulties you might find are:

1. What about feeding?

The chances are you have been told from every source out there that you must, must, must breastfeed, as it makes your baby healthier, smarter, stronger and faster to develop. Plus it will help you lose weight, promote bonding and be easier and cheaper than formula feeding. Although all of these pros are right, some are exaggerated (usually by women who find breastfeeding easy and have an endless supply of milk).

fact

What is true to say is that breastfeeding is good for your baby and for you, *if* you can do it, *if* your baby latches on easily and *if* you enjoy the process.

The reality is that plenty of women can't and don't like breastfeeding, usually because they haven't had the right kind of help, so no matter how much they try, either the baby won't latch on properly, or their nipples hurt too much or the baby cries so much that they give up and turn to formula.

The good news is there are plenty of ways to make breastfeeding easier and make the experience successful.

1. Ask for help and keep asking until you get it (see Resources for helplines). This means asking your midwife, health visitor, GP and even friends who have done it successfully for tips and advice. New mother forums on parenting sites can be really helpful in this area as well. Your midwife should be able to answer all your worries and show you how to hold and get your baby to latch on.
2. Give yourself a chance. Breastfeeding takes time to get the hang off and not every baby and mum takes to it like a duck to water. The more you try the more likely you are to get the hang of it. Bear in mind it can help to put a cushion under your arm to help support your baby, and sit in a quiet and peaceful room with the phone switched off so you don't have anything to stress you out.
3. If you're a true lazy girl/mum then bear in mind that breastfeeding is going to be your best friend because there

is no feed to mix up and carry round when you're out and about, no bottles to wash and sterilise and no having to go downstairs at night to heat up a bottle.

4. Being well informed is everything when it comes to breastfeeding so make sure you know the facts about latching on, how to tell if your baby is feeding correctly, and what to do if you have sore and painful breasts, as well as how to look after yourself when breastfeeding (see below).

Getting to grips with breastfeeding

If you do want to breastfeed it's a great thing that can make you both feel relaxed and happy, so here are the key points to know:

- Breastfeeding does burn an extra 500 calories per day, which can help you lose the 'baby fat' and helps your uterus contract back to its pre-pregnant size.
- Position is everything with breastfeeding. Turn your baby towards your breast and bring his nose in line with your nipple.
- The aim is to help your baby to get a good mouthful of breast. Never let your baby suckle on the nipple. Apart from this being painful, the baby gets the milk from squeezing the ducts around the nipple, not the nipple itself.
- Let your baby feed on demand in the first few weeks to get your milk supply established and when he feeds don't rush him. The first part of the feed is watery and quenches his thirst (known as foremilk); the second is

higher in calories and is called hindmilk. Together they make up the perfect feed.

- Always make a note of which breast you fed from last so you don't feel lopsided (you'll probably notice because the engorged full breast is the one you'll need to feed from next).

- Ask for help if you're struggling (see Resources) as there are plenty of places that can help you, usually at all hours of the day.

- Take it easy. Breastfeeding on demand is exhausting and if you rush about or rush feeds your milk may dry up or your baby will not feed properly.

- Be careful what you eat and drink while breastfeeding. Everything that goes through you goes into your breastmilk but also make sure you drink plenty of water to keep your supply steady.

- A newborn baby needs to be fed every two to three hours, but when you start breastfeeding it may be every hour. To get enough food, give your baby the chance to nurse for about 10–15 minutes at each breast.

- Always have a glass of water next to you. Breastfeeding is thirsty work for you.

If however, you have tried everything, asked for help and it still seems as if your baby cries all the time because he's hungry or you weep with anxiety every time you try to feed, or you suffer from continuous mastitis (painful swelling in the breast of a breastfeeding woman that may be caused by a blocked milk duct or an infection) then do yourself a favour and stop. Don't feel guilty or assume you're a bad mother, or that you have done something wrong, because you haven't.

As a mother, sometimes you have to think that what's good for you will be good for your baby. What's more, plenty of babies are bottle-fed and do just as well as breastfed babies.

fact

Babies can't digest solid food before six months, and the signs that they are ready are: they can stay in a sitting position with their head steady, reach out and grab food, and eat some of it themselves. Until then, keep giving them milk.

2. Wind/burp your baby

Babies often swallow air during feeds, which can make them feel terrible, as they don't yet know how to get rid of it. You can prevent this by winding your baby every 50ml (2fl oz) 90ml (3fl oz) if you bottle-feed, and each time you switch breasts if you breastfeed. To wind/burp your baby, hold your baby upright with her head on your shoulder. Support your baby's head and back while gently patting the back with your other hand. If that doesn't work, lay your baby face down on your lap. Support her head, making sure it's higher than her chest, and gently pat or rub her back.

Care for when baby is asleep

- Always place your baby on his back when he's asleep.
- Don't smoke or allow people to smoke around your baby.

- Remove loose bedding, pillows and stuffed toys from the sleep area so that they can't fall on your baby's face (your baby is too young to push them off).
- Take care when the baby is in your bed and don't let him sleep with you if either of you have been drinking.
- Make sure your baby isn't too hot and that the room is cool.
- Try using a dummy/pacifier to help him sleep, as this may help protect against SIDS.
- Let your baby sleep in your room until he is six months old.
- Be aware that most babies need a night feed until they are around 12 weeks. Some stop before this time and some go on for longer.

fact

Contrary to what some books say, breastfed babies need winding too.

3. Will it be love at first sight?

Bonding is the name given to the attachment that develops between parents and their baby. Studies show that the strong ties between parents and their baby is what helps foster a sense of security and positive self-esteem in a child and helps a child to develop. The problem is that while most babies are hardwired to bond immediately (mainly due to the fact that their survival depends on it), for parents it can be a lot harder. And although much is written about mothers and bonding, dads can also have a problem with it, partly because dads can't breastfeed and often have to go back to work fairly quickly after the birth.

What you need to know is this: bonding is rarely instantaneous. It is a process that grows through getting to know each other. And while it is love at first sight for some mums and their babies, for many women it takes much longer to bond. If this happens to you, it doesn't mean you don't love your baby but more that you simply don't feel a special attachment to your child yet. This can happen for many reasons:

- A traumatic delivery has left you exhausted.
- High expectations of what having a baby will be like and the response you'll get from your child (newborns don't actually do very much).
- The belief you should have bonded instantly and the ensuing guilt that you haven't.
- Having a boy when you wanted a girl, or vice versa.
- Feeling depressed in general.
- Relationship, family or financial problems.
- A baby who cries a lot, or won't feed or sleep.
- Being ill and separated from your child after birth.

4. How to bond

The good news is you can help to promote bonding by understanding how your baby attaches to you. Firstly, babies love to be touched and held (and, contrary to popular belief, you cannot 'spoil' a baby by holding them too much). This is one reason why skin-to-skin contact is so heavily promoted right after birth. Feeling your body so close to theirs is soothing and reassuring and helps them to feel secure. Try to hold your baby as much as possible and at the same time make eye contact with them and talk to them as you do this.

While it can feel hard to know what to say, try to remember your baby is not judging you in any way. So you can sing to them, chatter about what's on TV, and even read the newspaper to them and they will love it.

tip

If you feel embarrassed about chatting to a baby, try singing nursery rhymes or telling them a story.

What's important is the contact you're making, not what you say. Better still, just give them a running commentary of what you're doing, such as 'Now we're changing your nappy … now we're going upstairs' and so on.

Bonding also occurs with breastfeeding; although this is not always the case, so don't feel bad if it isn't happening to you. Bottle-fed babies bond just as well; studies show that babies respond to the smell and touch of their mothers, and to the fact that you're giving them what they need, not how you're doing it. Help yourself by:

- Looking after your baby as much as you can. You may feel afraid/worried or even unable to hold, feed and change her but the more you do it, the closer you will feel to your child.
- Talking to someone about how you feel. A health visitor or midwife can often be a good sounding board if you're afraid to admit your feelings to your partner or family.
- Understanding that in the future (once you have bonded) your child won't hold it against you.

• Thinking about your expectations of how you thought you'd feel as a mother. Sometimes it's this that holds us back from enjoying the reality of being a mum.

5. What should I do with a newborn?

Very young babies can only tolerate small periods of interaction, and like gentle and not rough play. This means playing with your baby in 10-minute spurts and doing small things like singing to him, turning a mobile on over his head or letting his eyes follow a rattle. At this age young babies also like play gyms they can look at, watching their reflections in mirrors, and soft rattles that make gentle noises. They also love being outdoors and seeing around them. So, basically anything you do with them will entertain them. This means you don't need expensive toys or visits to anywhere special. A simple trip to the park is enough, or even a visit to the supermarket.

A routine makes for a happy baby – and a happier you

Instead of thinking about what to do with your baby, think about bringing in a gentle routine to your lives. Babies love routines and will be happier if they know what's coming next, such as a nap at 10.00 a.m., lunch at 12.00 p.m., and so on. It will also make your life easier and more bearable if you know that there is a pattern to your day.

6. How can I stop my baby crying?

All babies cry. Why? Because it's the only way they can communicate with you and let you know something is up. The good news is that babies do not, contrary to popular belief, cry all the time (and if they do you should see your doctor to make sure they are OK). On the whole, babies cry for around two to three hours a day and not all at once. In time you'll be able to work out what's up and what each cry means. In the meantime, here is a crying checklist:

Does my baby need a feed? Being hungry is the most common reason why a baby will cry. The younger and smaller your baby is, the more likely it is that he is crying because he is hungry. Babies' tummies are small and most babies can't hold very much milk for long, so even if you feel you have just fed him, try giving him another feed. Other babies are just hungry babies and need to be fed more. Again, try upping the feed to see if it soothes him.

Is my baby too cold/too hot? Newborns get cold and too hot very quickly (remember it was the same temperature all the time inside your womb), so many will protest at a sudden temperature change. This happens the most when you change their nappies or if they get wet. Having said that, be careful not to get them too hot. Most babies need to wear one more layer of clothing than we do inside the house (more, obviously, when you go out).

fact

A baby can get too hot or too cold in an instant. Check whether your baby is too hot or too cold by feeling her stomach or neck (not forehead or feet and hands, which are often cold).

Does she need to a cuddle? Some babies need more cuddling than others and will cry until they are picked up. Ignore all 'experts' (and this includes family and partners) who tell you that by holding the baby too much you're either spoiling the baby or letting them manipulate you. Young babies do not know how to manipulate, all they know is what they need – that is: you, a cuddle, a feed, a change, or a sleep, and so on. The fact is, babies need physical contact to feel comforted.

Does he need a nap? Having said the above, your baby will also cry if he is over-stimulated; that is, held too much, picked up too much and played with too much. Although this often happens if you have too many visitors, it's important to learn to 'read' your baby's signals. If your baby cries when there are too many people around, and resists being picked up by others, take him into a quiet room where you can dim the lights and hold him and let him calm down.

Does she have colic? Colic is a condition that's characterised by inconsolable crying from late afternoon onwards. It usually starts from about three weeks and can last for up to four months. Doctors aren't sure what causes it; some people think it's muscle spasms caused by milk problems, and others by the intestines growing, and others believe it is wind. It's distressing to witness and hard to deal with, especially when you're tired. See your doctor for advice and help.

"I could never get my baby to stop crying in my arms, but what did work was putting him in front of the washing machine or taking him for a ride in his pushchair. I think the rhythmic motion and noise really helped soothe him."

Lisa, 32

fact

Babies who are breastfed also get colic, even though many experts say they don't.

7. How many guests and visitors should I have?

While it's natural that everyone wants to come to see your baby and shower you with gifts, people without children, and even people with children, can be too much in the early days, not only for you but your baby too. Being passed from relative to relative isn't pleasant for a young baby and can make a baby yell its head off if it goes on for too long or cause a contented baby to cry if it's routine is continually disrupted.

What's more, in the early weeks your baby is building up its immunity and so the less people you have around the less likely it is that your baby will catch a cold. On top of this, you need your rest, and rushing about making tea and keeping the house tidy can be the straw that breaks a new mum's back. So here's what you need to do:

- Ask friends not to come round when they are ill or their kids are.
- Don't wait on your friends and family when they come round; ask them to help make tea/coffee/lunch.
- Get friends to come round in two-hour slots – that's about enough for you and your baby.
- Never have more than two visitors at a time.
- When you have guests, keep to your baby's routine even if relatives complain.

- Breastfeed in a different room, it will help your baby feed better.
- Don't be afraid to put people off coming for a few weeks.
- Put your needs and that of your baby before what friends and family want.
- Don't overdo it. You may want the company, but having an open house for friends and family will make you ill when you have a new baby.

Life after birth – what now?

Apart from learning how to be a new parent and dealing with a very young baby, the other part of being a busy mum is getting to grips with the life change that will affect every part of your life from your body to your mindset. Adapting to your new role often means having to think about the old you and your old life and working out how you can merge these with the person you're becoming. It all sounds very touchy-feely, but it's a process that needs to be faced one way or another before potential problems emerge.

Problem 1: I can't bear being on my own all day

If you were a career girl, the chances are that up until now you have been used to a bustling, busy office where you had colleagues and friends to see and talk to daily and a schedule that made good use of your brain. Being at home with a baby, no matter how happy that baby makes you, doesn't detract from the fact that learning to be on your own and making your own schedule is hard.

"Every day felt like groundhog day. I used to cry when my husband went to work because the thought of having no one to talk to all day was just relentless."

Susie, 30

What's important to know is that getting used to being home all day is an adjustment that takes time. Although it can be lovely to not have to commute or get involved in office politics, feeling that life is happening outside your window without you can make you feel lonely. To help yourself, make sure you:

- Go out with your baby once a day, every day.
- Create a routine that breaks up your day into chunks you can deal with.
- See and make new mum friends with women who live near to you.
- Get changed out of your pyjamas – it may be comfy but it won't make you feel good if all you do is wear nightwear all week.
- Invite friends over during the day.
- Join mum forums and Internet sites so that you can email people in a similar situation to yourself.

Problem 2: I am tired *all* the time

Most mothers would agree that the worst thing about having a baby is the continuously disrupted sleep and the feeling of perpetual tiredness that never seems to go away. In fact it's easy to see why sleep deprivation is a form of torture, because being tired affects everything from how you think to how you perform tasks to how you feel about life. To help yourself:

- **Rest when the baby sleeps** So, don't rush about cleaning the house, emailing friends and calling your mum while your baby sleeps. Lie down, take a nap or just watch TV.
- **Go to bed earlier** This one can be hard, but in the early days when your baby is waking every three hours all night for a feed, it helps to hit the bed around 9.00 p.m. At least then you get in a few hours before the feeding process starts.
- **Ask for help** You may want to do it all on your own, but you don't have to if you have friends and family ready to step in.
- **Eat properly** Snacking on sugary food and fizzy drinks and caffeine will just increase your tiredness. If all else fails, prepare your lunch and snacks the night before, especially if you're breastfeeding.
- **Shop online** It will save you one big chore from your to-do list.
- **See your doctor for help** if the tiredness increases, even though your baby is sleeping through.

Problem 3: I have no me-time

As much as you may have a partner who helps, the brunt of childcare in the early weeks will always fall on the mother, especially if you're breastfeeding and on maternity leave. No matter how much you love your child, finding yourself unable to have a moment alone to think or to do what you want can be hard. If you were a very busy girl who loved what she did for a living, this aspect of new motherhood can feel soul-destroying. To help yourself:

- Get organised. Motherhood is easier when you have a routine, even if you're not a routine kind of girl. Best of all, babies love routines and your day will have more me-time space if you know when feeds, walks and naps are scheduled in.
- Have a night out with a friend. You may not feel like it, but it will re-energise your life.
- One of the most important things about 'me time' is regularity. What's important is not a weekend away but daily time alone. Try trading time with your partner: an hour to yourself reading the paper, for an hour when he can watch TV and so on.
- As much as you can, try taking your 'me-time', away from home. Even a walk alone in the park is good for you.
- Don't include showering or domestic chores as 'me-time'. Practise putting your needs at the top of your list once a day.
- Don't always wait for structured time. Seize 'me-time' whenever you can: when your baby is napping in the pushchair, read a book or when you're breastfeeding, watch a DVD.

Problem 4: I hate my post-pregnancy body

Apart from the 1 per cent of women who snap back into shape in the delivery room, most women hate their bodies post-pregnancy. Why? Well, for the last nine months, although you have had a growing bump, that bump has been nice and firm and solid. Now your baby is out, the bump is like a deflating balloon: wobbly, loose and, let's face it, fairly floppy. Add to this your breasts, which if you're breastfeeding are probably huge and if you're weaning or not breastfeeding are deflating into shapeless pockets. And all this before we talk about baby weight gain.

Before you smash all the mirrors in your house, bear a couple of things in mind. Firstly, pregnancy weight takes nine months to gain, so your body is going to take at least this time to get back into pre-pregnancy shape. Secondly, your uterus contracts slowly over four to six weeks and your stomach muscles are so stretched that your belly will feel soft and bloated. After six weeks have passed and you are given the go ahead by your doctor you can help speed things up with a healthy diet and exercise, although bear in mind that this takes time. Thirdly, the body stores fat during pregnancy to prepare for breastfeeding, so if you do breastfeed, you might loose some of that weight, but as you also need some 500–800 calories extra per day to produce the milk, you may find yourself eating more. The answer is to think about what you eat (whether you're pregnant or not). Help yourself by eating healthy foods over fast, sugary snacks so that you lose weight at a steady rate.

Simple ways to help yourself get back into shape

- Stock your cupboards with healthy food, such as fruit, nuts, crackers and low-fat cheese, and dump all the crisps, biscuits and cakes.

- Go for a long walk every day with your baby. Walking for 60 minutes a day burns 200–400 calories an hour (depending on how fast you walk).
- Don't take celebrity post-pregnancy advice – it's never realistic and never the whole truth.
- Be realistic about what you want to achieve and your time frame.
- Join a post-pregnancy fitness group and get professional advice on how to get back in shape effectively.
- Boost your self-esteem by reminding yourself of what your body has actually done over the last nine months!

Problem 5: All my clothes look awful

Apart from body anxieties, feeling frumpy, mumsy and downright dowdy, post-pregnancy is enough to make any new mum want to hide inside all day. This problem is directly related to the one above, and becomes a problem because maternity clothes tend to look better on a pregnant woman, not one with a deflating stomach, and pre-pregnancy clothes tend to look better on women who haven't just had a baby. The solution is to do a couple of things. Firstly, buy a few items that are in fashion. (Having been out of the fashion scene for nine months you're bound to feel frumpy.) It may seem like a waste of money, but new wardrobe staples will get you through this in-between stage and are essential to helping you feel and look good:

- Depending on your body, you can either opt for mid-maternity wear or a bigger size in normal clothes.

- Be sure to update your underwear too, as your bra size will have changed again, and the right bra size is essential if you want your clothes to look good. Granny pants (knickers with a hold-in panel) can also help you to feel better.
- Look after your overall appearance. A good haircut or facial will sometimes be all you need to refresh your look and make you feel a new and more stylish woman.
- Buy clothes that work on disguising the parts you hate. For instance, flared sleeves if you feel your upper arms are too big, a V-neck if you feel your breasts are taking over, and dark trousers or skirts to lengthen your look.
- If you're breastfeeding, bear in mind that your breasts will change size when they engorge (fill with milk) so buy tops that are made from stretchable fabrics (and which also give easy access).
- Buy a big scarf/pashmina – not only do they hide a multitude of sins but they are also excellent if you're breastfeeding in public and want to be discreet.

Problem 6: I have no time for my relationship

There's nothing like going from two to three to put a strain on a relationship. Apart from the fatigue factor, adjusting to being a family is hard on all sides. For starters, it can be hard to make time for each other, and resentment can easily grow if one of you feels the other isn't pulling their weight or is making no effort to understand how hard it is. On top of this, lack of sleep and stress about being new parents can make you snappy with each other and cause arguments that may once have been non-existent in your relationship.

"We'd been together for ten years before we had our son and hardly ever argued. Once we had Tom, we argued all the time and about everything. It was tough and I realised that we never argued before we had kids because we didn't have much to argue about. Now everything is an issue, from whose turn it is to do the night feed to who does more."

Karen, 34

The good news is that there are a multitude of things you can do to improve things, starting with talking together about the issues you are facing as new parents. Whether this is feeling cut off at home, jealous about the lack of attention or just fed up with the whole thing. Help yourself by:

- Listening as much as you speak. What is it your partner is trying to say and what is it that he wants?
- Making date time for each other, whether it's once a week or once a month. Remember, a date can be at home if you're reluctant to leave your baby.
- Getting intimate. If you have no energy for sex, make sure you keep kissing and hugging. Staying close can stop you feeling cut off from each other.
- Not taking over all the baby duties. Encourage your partner to bond with the baby for his sake as well as your child's (and don't police him when he's doing this).
- Praising each other's parenting skills. It can help to know someone thinks you're doing a good job.

- Scheduling time for sex. OK, so it's not spontaneous, but this doesn't mean it's going to be rubbish. Apart from the fact that you can mentally get ready for it, choosing a time when the baby is asleep and you have the energy means better sex all round.

Problem 7: I am nervous around my baby and scared to take him out

All new mothers are nervous around their babies. Even the mothers who used to run companies, do major surgery or deal with millions of pounds every day. Why? Well, because having a very young baby is terrifying; apart from the baby being small and vulnerable, you constantly worry that you're doing the wrong thing, or will drop him/accidentally bump him or hurt him. In time you'll see that babies are fairly durable, but until then, for your own sanity, you have to work on building up your confidence.

"I hated bathing my son. What no one ever tells you is how slippery the baby is and how they scream because they hate it. I used to get so jittery and nervous every time I did it I was practically in tears by the end."

Kelly, 30

The best way to deal with this problem is to face it head on. Like anything that makes you scared and nervous, you have to take it one step at a time. Start by:

- Making a list of the top ten things that scare you. For instance, going on public transport with the baby, bathing the baby, feeding the baby in public, driving with the baby, and so on. Then, every day make sure you do one thing on the list and keep doing it until the fear starts to diminish.
- Asking mum friends how they coped. You'll be amazed at the tricks other mums know and can pass on to you (also try the mum sites in Resources).
- Getting used to holding and playing with your baby. The more you interact with her the more confident you will feel handling her.
- If you're nervous when you're out and about with your baby, think of ways to make yourself feel more secure. Perhaps a pushchair that faces you as opposed to facing away, so that you can see your baby. Or ask a friend or relative to come with you.
- Seeking out baby-friendly places on the Internet in advance when you're going somewhere. Although most places always have baby changing facilities, many don't have highchairs or allow pushchairs in. Knowing where you're going before you venture out will put your mind at rest.
- Don't overwhelm yourself (or your baby). If you're not ready to do two weeks away in a foreign country, then don't do it. Make your life easy.

tip

If the fear and anxiety doesn't go away, see your doctor. Overwhelming anxiety and fear can be a sign of postnatal depression.

Problem 8: Am I getting postnatal depression (also known as postpartum depression)?

Having a history of depression, little or no support post-baby, and having to go through a traumatic birth can all make you more likely to get postnatal depression (PND); however, you can't talk yourself into it (or out of it), and if you do have it you shouldn't try to cope alone. Which is why it's important to be aware of the signs of PND and seek help as soon as you feel it's happening to you.

Being prepared is your best defence against PND: know what to expect and what to do post-baby if you feel depressed. Know who can help – your midwife, doctor, health visitor and a range of helplines (see Resources) – and know that PND can be treated (via antidepressants and counselling).

Postnatal depression symptoms

If you answer yes to any of the following, see your doctor for an expert diagnosis:

- Do you feel persistent sadness and numbness?
- Do you feel you are a 'bad' mother?
- Do you have distressing thoughts about yourself and your baby?
- Are you anxious or obsessive about your baby's health, welfare and safety?
- Do you feel unable to enjoy life, have a sense of humour and laugh like you did before having your baby?
- Do you feel 'not right in yourself' since the birth of your baby?
- Are you pretending everything is OK to everyone?
- Are you reluctant to pick up your baby when she cries?

Problem 9: I never, ever want another child!

You may never want another child, but if you're using your present experience as the reason why you're never having sex again, never mind getting pregnant or having a baby again, then the chances are you'll change your mind. Everyone feels that way in the early days, simply because they are exhausted, daunted and so busy they don't have time to breathe, but life with a child gets easier. Yes, different problems surface, but eventually you will get more sleep, you will have more me-time and you probably will want to get pregnant and do it all over again.

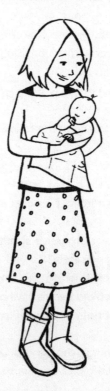

20 *ways*

to make life with a baby easier on yourself

1 Don't aim to be super-mum
Seeking perfection is the enemy of the lazy girl and busy mum – keep reminding yourself that your baby doesn't need you to be perfect; he just needs you to be yourself.

2 Don't be friends with competitive mums
Anyone who says, 'Oh you're not breastfeeding/teaching him his alphabet/encouraging him to talk' should be dumped immediately from your new friend list.

3 Set boundaries with friends
Especially with friends who call up for a chat at 11.00 p.m. or think you still have hours and hours to deal with their problems. Boundaries are what will make your life easier on all fronts.

4 Use your spare time wisely
Be selfish and put yourself first, whether that's using spare time to sit alone in a café and read a book, have a facial or go shopping alone. It doesn't need to be spent tidying up or meeting people you'd rather not see.

5 Go easy on the baby groups

As the weeks go on it will be clear what kind of groups your baby likes and needs. It's tempting to do everything to fill your time and meet new people, but remember, you don't have to do anything. There is plenty of time (and years) for your baby to become social.

6 Read up on child development

Not to work out if you have a child genius but so that you know that all babies and children progress differently. It doesn't matter if your baby isn't smiling yet and everyone else's is – she will eventually do it, because all children do.

7 Remind yourself it's a phase!

Going through a bad patch where your baby screams all the time, or won't sleep or just refuses to have his nappy changed? Well, rest assured it's just a phase. Meaning, it will pass – and sooner than you think!

8 Enjoy the here and now

As hard as it is with a newborn baby, don't wish it away. The baby phase passes in a blink of an eye, so enjoy it as much as you can.

9 Don't rush back to work

Even if you hate being on maternity leave, don't rush back to full-time work. Apart from the fact that your baby needs you, you need time to recover from the birth and to get to grips with your new role. Give yourself time to get used to it.

10 Exercise daily

Not only will it get you out of the house, but it will also give you more energy and help improve your body image. See Resources for ideas on what to do.

11 When in doubt, ask

Worried about a rash, a strange nappy or even what your baby is or isn't doing? Don't suffer in silence or fear, ask your doctor or health visitor for advice.

12 Go with your gut instinct

You know your baby best, because you are with your baby more than anyone else. So, if you are worried about your baby's development, an illness or something else entirely, always get a second opinion. Most good doctors will acknowledge that mum knows best.

13 Don't overpack when you go out

Your baby is the size of a small puppy, so why do you need to go out with a bag filled with 20 nappies, three feeds and four clean outfits? Less is more with babies on all fronts, from toys to clothes to what's in the changing bag.

14 Forget being a yummy mummy

As if there wasn't enough to be worried about, trying to be a yummy mummy (that is, a sexy and stylish mum) is something that you shouldn't bother with unless it just comes naturally.

15 Let go of your expectations

Suspend your expectations and accept your baby for the person she is. Don't think she should be sleeping through the night/eating more/being more social. Babies have their own time frame for doing things, let your baby be.

16 Take all the shortcuts you need

From online shopping to ready meals, to bought birthday cakes – if it makes your life easier, then it's the right decision.

17 Teach your baby a few tricks

If you're not breastfeeding, get your baby used to drinking milk at room temperature, then you don't need to heat bottles when you are out. Just add the powder and shake well!

18 Forget about mummy guilt

Whether you go back to work, stay at home, work from home or do a combination of all three, you will feel guilty. Lessen the guilt by reminding yourself you're working for your family, not just for fun.

19 Take a break

If all the crying, yelling and demanding is getting you down, step outside for five minutes and take some deep breaths – your baby will be fine and you'll return more able to cope.

20 Believe in yourself

Motherhood can seem daunting and overwhelming, so it pays to remind yourself why you're well equipped to deal with it. Write a list of all your best attributes and stick it to your fridge/mirror as a reminder when things get tough.

CHAPTER EIGHT

A–Z of pregnancy

If you're too busy to read the whole book at once, here's a lazy girl's glossary of essential pregnancy facts you really should know.

A is for antenatal

Also known as the pre-natal period, this is the time between conception and birth; that is, the long 40 weeks from getting pregnant to having your baby. Hence, antenatal classes, antenatal appointments and antenatal tests.

B is for breastfeeding

Breastfeeding is when you exclusively feed your baby with breast milk, and don't mix your feeds with formula (which is known as mixed feeding). Breastfeeding is a hotly debated subject with some experts saying women should exclusively breastfeed for six months, although this advice is not practical or realistic for everyone. Like everything, breastfeeding is a personal choice. Choosing not to breastfeed won't make you a bad mother or stop you bonding with your baby.

B is for Braxton Hicks

Braxton Hicks are sporadic contractions of the uterus that occur throughout pregnancy. They can be felt as a tightening or hardening at the front of the abdomen that lasts for a minute or so and are generally noticed mid pregnancy. Unlike 'real' labour contractions, Braxton Hicks tend to be irregular and disappear quite quickly.

Experts believe that Braxton Hicks contractions help to encourage the flow of blood to the placenta and to tone and soften the muscles of the uterus so as to support and protect the foetus.

C is for Caesarean

A Caesarean section is a medical procedure that involves cutting the abdomen and womb in order to deliver a baby. Although fewer women have their baby this way, opting instead for a normal vaginal delivery, figures for Caesareans are on the rise. There are many reasons a doctor might perform one, from a baby being in distress during delivery (known as an emergency C-section) to problems with the mother's health pre-labour or the position of the baby during labour. Post-op, it takes around six weeks for the abdominal tissue to heal from a C-section.

A small word about what's known as an elective Caesarean. This is where you can opt to have a Caesarean section, even though you don't need one, on a specific day around the time of your due date. This is a favourite of the celebrities who are supposedly 'too posh to push' and you may be given the option depending on the country in which you live and the type of healthcare you have opted for (in this case private).

However, beware if you're considering it. A Caesarean, elective or otherwise, is an operation and not the easy option. You may not have to suffer labour pains, but the recovery period is longer and tougher, due to stitches that make it painful to do everything from drive to picking your baby up.

C is for colostrum

This is the first breast milk to appear after a baby is born, and it is what your baby drinks before your milk supply comes in (usually two days after birth). Colostrum is thick and yellow, rich in proteins, minerals and antibodies and also works as a laxative.

D is for doula

Doula (pronounced 'doola') is a Greek word meaning 'woman servant or caregiver'. It now refers to an experienced woman who offers emotional and practical support to a woman (or couple) before, during and after childbirth. Birth doulas are trained and experienced in childbirth, although they are not trained midwives, so they are there to support the mother, not to give clinical advice. In some countries a doula is always present, in others you have to hire them privately.

E is for energy

Energy during pregnancy is an elusive thing. One moment you'll feel so exhausted that even walking down the stairs needs a 10-minute sofa recovery break, the next you'll feel as if you could run a marathon (although don't try it!). Much has to do with which trimester you're in, the first trimester and third being the worst for energy, the second being the best. Energy during pregnancy is also dependent on a few other factors that work in your favour, even when you're not pregnant, such as: drinking enough water during the day (vital during pregnancy when your body sucks up every ounce in your body), resting when you're tired and eating well.

E is for episiotomy

This is a surgical incision through the perineum made to enlarge the vagina and assist childbirth. In the past, up to 90 per cent of women in labour in the UK had episiotomies, but doctors now believe that they're not of great benefit and are unnecessary for most women, except when the baby is in distress or the mother is having a forceps delivery.

F is for flatulence

Rest assured, a large amount of bottom wind is completely normal during pregnancy and has much to do with the way your digestive system slows down during the pregnancy process. Food tends to sit around in your intestine for longer than usual to make sure your body can extract all the vitamins from it. So, the food ferments, festers and eventually escapes partially as gas. Try not to stress about it – like everything else in pregnancy, it's just a phase.

G is for growing bumps

Pregnancy bumps are weird things. Some people show right from the start, others have less of a bump at the front and show more from the side, and others don't show in the morning but always show at night. Whatever your growing bump decides to do, rest assured that in the beginning it will suddenly seem as if it has appeared overnight (and some actually do). So, remember that bump size and shape depend on various things. With your first baby, you're likely to have a neat bump, as the stomach muscles are tight, but the more children you have, the more lax your muscles become. Your bump may be more spread out or bigger because the muscles aren't holding in the baby so well.

Bump size also depends on how much fluid you've got inside and the way your baby is laying. It might also depend on your stature and posture.

H is for pregnancy hair

If you're one of the lucky ones, being pregnant means that your hair is shinier, thicker and more gorgeous than ever. This is because pregnancy causes more of your hair to enter into the resting phase, resulting in the appearance of thicker hair; that is, your hair doesn't fall out. Yet, for others, this extra production of hormones not only increases the amount of hair on their head but it also causes a bout of excessive hair growth. If you're very unlucky, being pregnant could mean that you have more body hair and the hair on your head is actually dryer, duller and more lifeless than before. Whichever way it goes, blame your hormones.

I is for indigestion

Indigestion is the name often given to a number of symptoms, including heartburn, regurgitation (food coming back up from the stomach), bloating and nausea, and vomiting. Half of all women experience indigestion at some point during their pregnancy, with the risk of indigestion increasing as the baby develops. This is mainly due to changes that occur in the body during pregnancy, such as rising levels of hormones and increased pressure on the abdomen from the foetus. These changes can often result in acid reflux, when stomach acid flows back up from the stomach into the oesophagus. Good news is that your GP can prescribe you something to ease the pain. Also, sitting up after you eat helps, and when you sleep make sure your head is raised (at least 15cm (6in) higher than usual) and this will stop acid flowing back into your throat as you sleep.

I is for induction

Induction is when your labour is started artificially either because you have gone over your due date or there is something wrong with either your health, the baby's health or the pregnancy. Your waters may be artificially broken in the hope that this will start labour, a 'sweep' may be done of your cervix by your doctor and you will be given a drug (an artificial version of the hormone oxytocin, which brings on labour) to start your contractions.

K is for Kegel

Kegel exercises, also called pelvic floor exercises, help strengthen the muscles that support the uterus, bladder and bowels – something that is vital during pregnancy, as this area is put under strain by the growing weight of your baby. Pregnant women who perform Kegel exercises develop the ability to control their muscles during labour and delivery. But most important of all is that toning all of these muscles will also minimise a common problem during and after pregnancy: bladder leaks. The best thing about Kegel exercises is that they can be done anywhere, and no one knows you're doing them.

L is for labour

They call it labour for a reason, because it is hard work. This doesn't mean it's excruciating, horribly painful and the worst thing ever, neither does it mean you won't be able to do it or will need to be zonked out to get through it. What's important is that you are realistic and also fully informed from the right sources about what labour is really all about! Other mums aren't always the right source for this information, as they will tend to give you a very subjective picture. Antenatal classes, your midwife and your doctor are the people who can advise you the most.

L is for lochia

This is a normal vaginal discharge that lasts for several weeks after the birth of a child and is the body's way of discharging the lining of the womb following the birth. Lochia is initially bright red, then becomes pinkish, and eventually yellowish or white.

M is for midwife

A midwife is a specialist who is qualified to give total care to you and your baby during pregnancy, labour and after the baby is born.

Midwives are the only professionals concerned solely with maternity care, and the only other people legally allowed to deliver babies are doctors, who need not have had specialist training in this field.

M is for morning sickness

A slightly misguided term because if you have morning sickness – and not all women do – it tends to happen, morning, noon and night, although for some women it is worse in the morning. It occurs in the first half of pregnancy; feeling sick and/or nauseated is very common and brought about by the hormonal changes taking place in the body and by an imbalance in blood sugar (it tends to happen more when you haven't eaten, which is ironic, because you don't want to eat when you have morning sickness). Most experts agree it's a good sign that the body is taking to the pregnancy. Small comfort I know.

N is for normal

While other mums and some experts are fond of saying that most effects are normal during pregnancy, it's worth pointing out that you need to be informed during pregnancy so you know what's normal and what isn't. Not only for the sake of your health but that of your pregnancy. For instance, it's normal to have morning sickness but not so normal to vomit so much you can't keep hydrated or move out of bed for weeks. It's normal to have itchy skin during pregnancy, but not be so itchy that you feel ill. In rare cases, severe itchiness in your third trimester can be a sign of a serious liver problem called obstetric cholestasis. In this case the itchiness is very widespread and often includes itching of the hands and feet.

O is for obstetrician

An obstetrician is a doctor who specialises in caring for pregnant women through childbirth and delivery. Depending on where you live you probably won't see an obstetrician until labour and only be checked by a midwife at your appointments. This is because women with complicated or difficult pregnancies make up a majority of an obstetrician's work. If you're not seeing one, rest assured all is fine.

P is for perineum

It's likely you've never heard of this before, but the perineum is the small stretch of skin between the vagina and rectum. Some experts, such as midwives and childbirth advisors, advise doing what's known as a perineal massage on this area during the latter stages of pregnancy. They feel it may help stretch the perineum in preparation for childbirth, and minimise stinging and tearing (see T for tears) when the baby's head passes through the vaginal opening. The suggested technique is to insert the thumbs or index fingers into the vagina, press downward toward the rectum, and then slide the fingers across the bottom and up the sides of the perineum.

P is for premature birth

Premature means that a baby is born several weeks earlier than your 'due date'. Most women have their babies between

37 and 42 weeks. The due date (EDD, or expected date of delivery) is calculated at 40 weeks. So, technically any baby born before the 37th completed week of pregnancy is termed premature. There are certain factors that may increase your likelihood of having a pre-term baby. These include illness during pregnancy, your health pre-pregnancy, a multiple pregnancy, and foetal problems, such as reduced growth and smoking.

P is for postnatal

The time following delivery until six weeks after birth is known as the postnatal period, a time when you will be checked regularly by midwives and doctors to make sure your body is recovering properly from the trauma of childbirth. After this period you are usually given the all-clear to exercise, have sex and generally go about your normal everyday life.

Q is for questions

While none of us like to look stupid, when you're pregnant it pays to ask questions and keep asking questions if you're confused, worried or generally in the dark about what's supposed to happen and why. That's not just about tests and delivery, but also about the day-to-day part of being pregnant. People to ask questions include: midwives, GPs, consultants, helplines (see Resources), other mums-in-the-know. Places to research queries: valid websites (see Resources) and pregnancy books. Pregnancy and parenting forums are especially good (see Resources), as it's unlikely you'll ever have a problem that another mum hasn't already gone through.

R is for rest

A pregnant woman needs more sleep and rest than she does when she's not pregnant. In most cases, eight to ten hours of sleep a night will help you feel better. Of course, this is not always practical, especially if you're unable to sleep or have no time to rest during the day because you're working. The way round this is to ensure you do rest when you have the time. In most cases this means less socialising, and more downtime. It sounds dull but it will pay off in the end, especially during labour when you need all the energy you can get.

S is for stretch marks

Around 75–90 per cent of women get stretch marks when they are pregnant, due to the skin stretching as you gain weight in the pregnancy. They usually appear as pinkish (or sometimes angry red or purple) lines on your abdomen, inside your legs, thighs and hips. Even if you rub oil or cream religiously into your skin, it's unlikely you'll avoid them. What's more, unfortunately stretch marks are permanent, although they do fade after your baby is born.

T is for tears

A perineal tear is a rip in the skin and muscles between the vagina and the rectum that usually happens during childbirth if the baby comes out too quickly (one reason why you should stop pushing if your midwife tells you to stop). If a woman appears to be at risk of a perineal tear during delivery, an episiotomy may be performed. This is a surgical cut that enlarges the area. Midwives now try very hard to avoid doing episiotomies, because they can cause problems with pain and healing post-delivery.

U is for uterus

You may never have thought about your uterus, and really who does? But it's important to understand its function during pregnancy. The uterus is made of smooth muscle lined with glands. The muscle is designed to contract during labour, orgasm and menstruation. Think of the uterus as a baby incubator. It expands to accommodate your baby and also works with the placenta to supply the baby with nutrients. When it's time for the baby to be born, the uterus contracts to expel the baby and the placenta and then the uterine muscle fibres start to contract, and over the course of eight to ten weeks the uterus shrinks back down again to just a little bigger than it was before you got pregnant.

V is for vaginal discharge

During pregnancy, it's very common to experience increased vaginal discharge. Most causes are fairly normal and what you are noticing is simply leucorrhoea – a mild-smelling milky fluid or discharge – caused by increased blood flow to the area around the vagina. For some women the discharge increases as you approach labour and can be quite heavy. In fact, an increase and thickening in your discharge towards the end of pregnancy may be a sign that you are approaching labour. If your discharge is foul smelling, itchy or worrying in any way see your GP to get it checked out.

V is for vitamin K

Vitamin K is a substance that is naturally present in the body that plays an important part in helping blood to clot. At birth, a baby is born with very low stores of this vitamin, which are then quickly used up over the first few days of life. This leaves a baby vulnerable to a rare condition that affects 1 in 10,000 babies, known as vitamin K deficiency bleeding (VKDB). As a result, medical advice is that levels of vitamin K should be increased for the first few weeks of life to offer protection until a baby starts to produce its own vitamin K stores, which will then minimise the risk of this condition. Your baby can be given this orally or via an injection, although you get to choose the method.

W is for water births

These days most hospital delivery suites offer the option of a birthing pool for a water birth, as research has found water can reduce the need for pain relief during labour and help avoid assisted labour; however, it depends where you live and which hospital you're going to as to whether you'll be allowed to actually give birth in the water (many hospitals just use it during the first stage of labour to help ease contractions). At home, you can hire a birthing pool and with the consent of your midwife and doctor give birth in it, as long as there are no complications in the pregnancy.

X is for X-ray

While you're pregnant, you should avoid having an X-ray if possible. If it's essential, your doctor will assess whether the benefits of treatment outweigh the low risk of having an X-ray.

They may also consider using another imaging method instead, such as an ultrasound scan. X-rays during pregnancy do not increase the risk of miscarriage or cause problems in the unborn baby such as birth defects, physical or mental development problems; however, repeated exposure to radiation can damage the body's cells, which can increase the risk of cancer developing. X-rays during pregnancy carry a very small risk that exposing the unborn baby to radiation could cause cancer to develop during their childhood.

Y is for you

Sometimes it's easy to forget in pregnancy that what you think and want is as important as what someone else says you should do. Always listen to your gut instinct and don't let yourself be led into something that you don't feel is right for you, whether that's choosing or not choosing pain relief, breastfeeding or even exercising during pregnancy. Make what's known as an informed choice (research it and then decide for yourself) and you'll make the right decision for you and your baby.

Z is for zzzzzz

It's what you need the most of during pregnancy but what also becomes elusive the more pregnant you become. This is because the increasing size of the foetus can make it hard to find a comfortable sleeping position, but common physical symptoms also interfere with sleep as well:

- **The need to pee** Your kidneys are working harder to filter the increased volume of blood (30–50 per cent more than you had before pregnancy) moving through your body, and this filtering process results in more urine. Plus, as your baby grows and the uterus gets bigger, the pressure on your bladder increases. This means more trips to the bathroom, day and night. The number of night trips may be greater if your baby is active at night.
- **An increased heart rate** Your heart rate increases during pregnancy to pump more blood, and as more of your blood supply goes to the uterus, your heart will be working harder to send sufficient blood to the rest of your body, making it hard to relax.
- **Leg cramps, restless leg syndrome and backache** Pains in your legs or back are caused by the extra weight you're carrying. During pregnancy, the body also produces a hormone called relaxin, which helps prepare the body for childbirth. One of the effects of relaxin is the loosening of ligaments throughout the body, making pregnant women less stable and more prone to cramps and pain, especially at night.

Resources

Information for pregnancy and motherhood

UK

Birth, pregnancy and parenthood sites

Ask a Baby. Website: www.askbaby.com. Pregnancy
   information
Ask a Mum. Website: www.askamum.co.uk. Advice,
   information and mum tips on pregnancy, birth and
   babies
Babyworld. Website: www.babyworld.co.uk. Conception,
   pregnancy and birth
Bounty. Website: www.bounty.com. A wealth of
   information on pregnancy and babies
Babycentre. Website: www.babycentre.co.uk. Pregnancy,
   baby and toddler health information

MIDIRS, Midwives Information and Resource Service.
Website: www.choicesforbirth.org and www.midirs.org

Midwives Online. Website: www.midwivesonline.com. Ask a
midwife service

Mothers 35 Plus. Website: www.mothers35plus.co.uk.
Advice and information for older mums

Mumsnet. Website: www.mumsnet.com. Parenting
community with the aim to make parents' lives easier by
pooling knowledge, experience and support

National Childbirth Trust. Website: www.
nctpregnancyandbabycare.com. Offers antenatal and
postnatal courses, local support, breastfeeding support
and information to help parents

Netmums. Website: www.netmums.com. A local network
for mums offering a wealth of information on both a
national and local level

NHS Pregnancy information. Website: www.NHS.uk/
pregnancy

Pregnancy miscellaneous

NHS Pregnancy Smoking Helpline. Tel.: 0800 169 0 169
Lines open: 12.00 noon to 9.00 p.m. Website: www.
givingupsmoking.co.uk

Foods Standard Agency. Website: www.eatwell.gov.uk/
agesandstages/pregnancy

Stylish Maternity Wear

Babes with Babies. Website: www.babeswithbabies.com

Blooming Marvellous. Website: www.bloomingmarvellous.co.uk

Crave. Website: www.cravematernity.co.uk

Fun Mum. Website: www.funmum.com

Isabella Oliver. Website: www.isabellaoliver.com

Jo Jo Maman Bebe. Website: www.jojomamanbebe.com

Maternity Exchange. Website: www.maternityexchange.
co.uk

Picchu. Website: www.picchumaternity.com

Seraphine. Website: www.seraphine.com

Yummy Mummy. Website: www.yummymummymaternity.
co.uk

Underwear websites

www.bras4mums.co.uk

www.figleaves.com

www.hermama.com

Breastfeeding

NHS Breastfeeding Help. Website: www.breastfeeding.nhs.uk

Breastfeeding Network. Website: www.
breastfeedingnetwork.org.uk. An independent source of
support and information for breastfeeding women

La Leche. Website: www.laleche.org.uk. Helping mothers
to breastfeed through mother-to-mother support,
encouragement, information

Beauty

Green Baby. Website: www.greenbaby.co.uk

Liz Earle. Website: www.lizearle.com

Mama Baby Bliss. Website: www.mamababybliss.com
Mama Mio. Website: www.mamamio.com
Mum Stuff. Website: www.mumstuff.co.uk

Bags

Babes with Babies. Website: www.babeswithbabies.com
Happy Bags. Website: www.happybags.co.uk
Pink Lining. Website: www.pinklining.co.uk

Finances

National Debtline. Tel.: 0808 808 4000, website: www.
nationaldebtline.co.uk
Maternity Benefits. Website: www.dwp.gov.uk/publications/
specialist-guides/technical-guidance/ni17a-a-guide-to-
maternity
Maternity Rights, website: www.direct.gov.uk/en/Parents/
Moneyandworkentitlements/WorkAndFamilies/
Pregnancyandmaternityrights/index.htm
Health in Pregnancy Grant
Website: http://www.direct.gov.
uk/en/MoneyTaxAndBenefits/
BenefitsTaxCreditsAndOtherSupport/
Expectingorbringingupchildren/index

HM Revenue & Customs Helplines:
Child Benefit: 0845 302 1444
Child Benefit Northern Ireland: 0845 603 2000
Tax Credits: 0845 300 3900
Tax and Benefits Confidential: 0845 608 6000

Antenatal and postnatal fitness

Bump to Babe. Website: www.bumptobabe.co.uk
Mummies and Buggies. Website: www.mummiesandbuggies.
co.uk
Pushy Mothers. Website: www.pushymothers.com

Help for Labour

British Acupuncture Council. Website: www.acupuncture.
org.uk
Doulas. Website: www.doula.org.uk
Home Births. Website: www.homebirth.org.uk
The Society of Homeopaths. Website: www.homeopathy-
soh.org
Hypnobirthing. Website: www.hypnobirthing.co.uk
Independent midwives. Website: www.
independentmidwives.org.uk
TENS machine. Website: www.maternitytens.com
The Good Birth Company, water births and hiring pools.
Website: www.thegoodbirth.co.uk

Post-birth Help

Cry-sis. Tel.: 08451 228 669, website: www.cry-sis.org.uk.
Help if you have a crying, sleepless and demanding baby
Parentline Plus. Tel.: 0808 800 2222, website: www.
parentlineplus.org.uk
Postnatal Illness/Depression.Website: www.pni.org.uk
Postnatal Depression. Website: www.mind.org.uk

Australia

Birth, pregnancy and babies

Australian Breastfeeding Association.Website: www.
  breastfeeding.asn.au
Babycenter. Website: www.babycenter.com.au
Belly Belly. Website: www.bellybelly.com.au
Birth.com. Website: www.birth.com.au
Home births. Website: www.homebirthaustralia.org
Kidspot. Website: www.kidspot.com.au
Nine Months. Website: www.ninemonths.com.au
Pregnancy Australia. Website: www.pregnancy.com.au
Queen Bee. Website: www.queenbee.com.au. Maternity
  clothes

Canada

Birth, pregnancy and babies

Babycenter. Website: www.babycenter.ca
Breastfeeding Canada. Website: www.breastfeedingcanada.ca
Canadian Parents. Website: www.canadianparents.com

New Zealand

Birth, pregnancy and babies

Home Birth. Website: www.homebirth.org.nz
Hot Milk Lingerie. Website: www.hotmilklingerie.co.nz

iParenting. Website: www.iparentingcanada.com
La Leche. Website: www.lalecheleague.org.nz
Natural Pregnancy. Website: www.pregnancy.health-info.org
Oh Baby. Website: www.ohbaby.co.nz
Parent Centres. Website: www.parentscentre.org.nz

South Africa

Birth, pregnancy and babies

Birth Works. Website: www.birthworks.co.za. Information
on natural birth
Doulas. Website: www.doulas.co.za
Fit Pregnancy. Website: www.fitpregnancy.co.za
La Leche League. Website: www.llli.org/SouthAfrica.html.
Breastfeeding
Postnatal Depression Support Association. Website: www.
pndsa.co.za

Index